W9-CFC-440

HOW FAST WILL YOU LOSE WEIGHT?

Research results in the Vanderbilt Program show that women will average a loss of approximately two-thirds of a pound a day for twenty-one days on the Rotation Diet. Some women will lose as much as a pound a day. Men may lose even more.

Many individuals lose two to three inches around the waist and buttocks in just three days, and can be one or two dress or pants sizes smaller in three weeks or less.

Thus, while the Rotation Diet is designed to help people who are significantly overweight, it is also the perfect diet for everyone who has struggled with the last five or ten pounds that stand between them and their most desirable weight.

With other diets, you soon begin to feel so deprived, and weight loss becomes so frustratingly slow, you just quit in disgust. Not so with the Rotation Diet. The rotation is the key to your success. Even if you have seventy-five pounds to lose, the Rotation Diet is the surest way to get that weight off easily and quickly—and keep it off.

Bantam Books by Martin Katahn
Ask your bookseller for the books you have missed

THE ROTATION DIET
THE T-FACTOR DIET

The Rotation Diet™

Martin Katahn, Ph.D.
DIRECTOR OF THE VANDERBILT
WEIGHT MANAGEMENT PROGRAM
AT VANDERBILT UNIVERSITY

BANTAM BOOKS
NEW YORK • TORONTO • LONDON • SYDNEY • AUCKLAND

*This edition contains the complete text
of the original hardcover edition.*
NOT ONE WORD HAS BEEN OMITTED.

THE ROTATION DIET
*A Bantam Book / published by arrangement with
W. W. Norton & Company, Inc.*

PUBLISHING HISTORY

*W. W. Norton edition published May 1986
Bantam edition / May 1987*

*All rights reserved.
Copyright © 1986 by Katahn Associates, Inc.
Author photograph copyright © 1987 by Dennis Wolf.
Cover design by Walter Harper.
Library of Congress Catalog Card Number: 86-8341.
No part of this book may be reproduced or transmitted
in any form or by any means, electronic or mechanical,
including photocopying, recording, or by any information
storage and retrieval system, without permission in
writing from the publisher.
For information address: W. W. Norton & Company, Inc.,
500 Fifth Avenue, New York, New York 10110.*

*If you purchased this book without a cover you should be aware that
this book is stolen property. It was reported as "unsold and
destroyed" to the publisher and neither the author nor the publisher
has received any payment for this "stripped book."*

ISBN 0-553-27667-0

Published simultaneously in the United States and Canada

*Bantam Books are published by Bantam Books, a division of Bantam Double-
day Dell Publishing Group, Inc. Its trademark, consisting of the words
"Bantam Books" and the portrayal of a rooster, is Registered in U.S. Patent
and Trademark Office and in other countries. Marca Registrada. Bantam
Books, 1540 Broadway, New York, New York 10036.*

PRINTED IN THE UNITED STATES OF AMERICA

OPM   22   21   20   19

Contents

Acknowledgments

I am greatly indebted to my many colleagues and students, who, from the start of the Vanderbilt Weight Management Program ten years ago, have contributed so much to the advances we have made in helping overweight persons. Without their help, the Rotation Diet would never have been created.

To begin with, it was my former student Dr. Gordon Kaplan who named the program when he recruited participants for his dissertation study on the factors that lead to long-term success in weight management. At that time, Dr. Kenneth Wallston joined us and assumed primary responsibility for the research component of the program. More recently, Dr. David Schlundt has collaborated in the development of our analysis of eating and activity problem areas, and in the design of our steps to weight-management mastery that form the basis for Chapters 9 through 11 of *The Rotation Diet*. Dr. Craig Heim, director of the Center for Health Promotion in the Vanderbilt Medical School, supervised the medical research that disclosed some of the health benefits associated with the Rotation Diet.

Another former student, Dr. Mark McMinn, contributed greatly with his studies of the biochemical factors that underlie the problem of obesity. Three of my present graduate students, Ruth Daby, Tracy Sbrocco, and Crystal Sulyma, are involved in implementing the Rotation Diet in the Vanderbilt Program and they have contributed to the development of the material in Chapters 9 through 11.

Our nutrition consultant, Rachel Willis, R.D., helped in the design of the Alternate Menus for the Rotation Diet that appear in Chapter 12. Her menus and recipes help me illustrate that eating nutritiously on a weight-reduction and weight-maintenance diet does not have to be boring, nor does it require an intolerable amount of deprivation. Thanks to CAMDE for supplying Nutri-Calc for performing our nutritional analyses; and thanks to our master baker, Joyce Weingartner, for creating the unique bread recipes that you will find in Chapter 6.

I want to express my special appreciation to the one person who keeps the entire Vanderbilt Weight Management Program on track by coordinating all of our efforts: my associate director, Summer Davis. In addition to her administrative skills, her own personal experience and understanding of the special problems that women face in managing their weight and her knowledge of how those problems are intertwined with other aspects of their lives enrich us all and contribute to our ability as leaders.

I don't know what I did to deserve them, but I have a very special family. Words can do little to express my love and appreciation, first, for being so supportive when I lost 75 pounds twenty-two years ago, second, for helping me maintain an environment that keeps it all off, and, third, for the joy they take in helping me create and test the interesting and delicious recipes for this and my other books. This time, in particular, my daughter, Terri, reviewed the first draft of everything I wrote, and helped design and write the recipes themselves.

Once again, just as he has in my two previous books, my editor at W. W. Norton, Starling Lawrence, provided invaluable critical advice in helping me write comprehensibly. In this instance, it was the difficult job of translating the clinically supervised Rotation Diet, just as we use it in the Vanderbilt Program, into book form. In addition, many others at W. W. Norton, and their friends, jumped in to test the diet as it was presented in the manuscript, to make sure we had succeeded. These included Iva Ashner, Linda Corrente, Dierdre Dolan, Jeannie Luciano, and Fran Rosencrantz, among many others. They provided the first, long-distance, daily reports of people trying the Rotation Diet on their own, and they gave us invaluable advice on how to present the program as simply and as understandably as possible. Their efforts have helped make *The Rotation Diet* easy to use. And their reward was the loss of an average of 11.5 pounds each. I would also like to thank Andy Marasia of the production department and Debra Makay of the editorial department at W. W. Norton.

As always—and I hope it goes on forever—my super agents,

Arthur and Richard Pine, have taken charge of every possible detail that could make an author's life less complicated. From the very beginning, when I first tried to tell the truth about the problems that overweight persons face and to explain what it really takes to manage your weight, the Pines, together with Starling Lawrence, have believed in the value of my work when others did not think the truth had "commercial value." Their support and boundless enthusiasm are truly appreciated.

And thanks again to my friends at Tandy for making sure that my computer, the Tandy 1200HD, never left me in the lurch during the writing of this book. The only time that I had a problem, when my keyboard decided it no longer wished to communicate with my computer, it took but one phone call and I had a replacement keyboard in my hands within twenty minutes, loaned to me while my own was sent in for repairs. I wish that every manufacturer and retailer of every mechanical and electronic device were as concerned about the needs of their customers as the folks at Tandy have been for mine throughout the many years that I have used their products.

Preface

As the paperback edition of *The Rotation Diet* goes to press, it seems appropriate to bring readers up to date on the success of the diet and to explain some changes that you can make in the daily menus that make it easier to use without decreasing its effectiveness.

First, thousands of reports have already flowed into our offices (see page 234) and these reports offer convincing evidence that the Rotation Diet can provide you, as a reader, with both the inspiration *and the instruction* you need to achieve permanent weight management. The Rotation Diet and Activity Program "feels good," and it provides the big payoff in terms of quick weight loss and effective maintenance that can motivate you to lose all the weight you need to lose and then keep it off.

Second, we have learned a great deal from the experience of people who have used the diet and found that they can be successful with certain deviations from the rather strict guidelines that I laid down in the original version. In the original version, unlimited free vegetables were limited to a list of 13 (see page 39). All vegetables in this list have fewer than 10 calories per half cup. In addition, the recommendation was made that the dieter limit his or her choice of safe fruit to just one variety rather than to a larger number. This guideline was established to prevent possible overeating on fruit snacks, which might interfere with the speed of weight loss.

Experience has shown that just about any fresh vegetable can be used in unlimited quantities with any of the meals on any day of the diet in order to be sure that you never leave the table hungry. Popular favorites, in addition to those listed on page 39, have been broccoli, tomatoes, carrots, mushrooms, all sorts of greens, cabbage (regular varieties as well as Chinese), and even onions! While these vegetables tend to average about 25 calories per half cup, the few extra calories do not seem to slow weight loss and the inclusion of this additional variety makes the diet much more interesting and satisfying. Perhaps the reason all vegetables seem to work, without impeding the loss of weight, is that they contain a lot of fiber (fiber is largely not digested) and a lot of water, which makes it hard to overeat.

Similarly, many people have found that they can achieve success more easily and comfortably if they vary their safe fruit, alternating among several rather than just one (see pages 39–41). There is no question that having only one choice of fruit as a snack (different fruits are recommended as part of the meal plans) can get boring—and when you get bored with your choice of safe fruit as a snack you may be more likely to revert to those dense-calorie foods that keep you fat. So, I have relaxed my recommendation—feel free to use a variety of safe fruits (other than avocado, which is very high in calories) for snacking. Have the tastiest available as they come into season, and you will find it much easier to avoid the candy, chips, and peanut butter crackers!

And remember, if you will just continue to substitute fresh fruit, any fruit, about 60 or 70 percent of the time when you might ordinarily eat high-calorie snacks or desserts after you reach your desirable weight, you will be taking a giant step toward permanent weight management.

Third, in the original version of the diet, my colleagues and I tried to maximize its nutritional value, even on the lowest calorie days, but still preserve palatability and variety. For example, within the grain group of foods we alternate recommending whole-grain breads, crackers, and breakfast cereals. This resulted in a diet that on the lowest calorie days was borderline concerning nutrients. You can remedy this situation by substituting a fortified cereal with skim or low-fat milk for breakfast, or for any other meal in place of bread or crackers. Many ready-to-eat breakfast cereals are fortified with from 25 to 100 percent of the Recommended Dietary Allowances of 10 to 13 different nutrients, including zinc, vitamin D, and iron (check the labels), and when eaten with milk will also significantly increase your intake of calcium.

I personally prefer cold breakfast cereals with a moderate to high amount of dietary fiber (from 2 to 5 grams per serving) and among my favorites are 40% Bran Flakes, Raisin Bran, Cracklin' Oat Bran, and Corn Bran. My wife prefers the very high fiber content of Bran Buds (8 grams per serving). Cereals with greater amounts of fortification than the ones I have just mentioned include Special K, Total, Product 19, and Just Right. These cereals are low in fiber, but you can increase the fiber content of any cereal by adding ½ cup of fresh fruit or a few teaspoons of All Bran. And, if you desire more variety in breakfast cereals, try sampling a number of the different ones that I have mentioned, or mixing them together—they are very different in taste and texture.

Although the inclusion of fortified breakfast cereals will significantly increase the nutritional value of the diet on its lowest calorie days, I still recommend a vitamin and mineral supplement for anyone who will use the Rotation Diet repeatedly in order to lose a large amount of weight.

I encourage you to try the Rotation Diet with the increased flexibility that I have just suggested. I think you will enjoy it more and perhaps be even more successful than you would have been had you used the less flexible version.

1

Introduction

HOW FAST WILL YOU LOSE?

"How fast can I lose weight on your diet?"

"Will I ever be able to eat like a normal human being and not gain weight?"

These are easily the most frequently asked questions on the lips of persons about to enter the Vanderbilt Weight Management Program, and they are among the first questions I am asked as I go around the country speaking on the topic of weight management.

Finally, after twenty-two years of personal experience maintaining my own weight loss of 75 pounds and ten years of work helping others lose weight in the Vanderbilt Program, I am able to give answers that will satisfy everyone who has 10, 20, 50, even 75 pounds of weight to lose:

Research results with participants in the Vanderbilt Program show that women will average a loss of approximately *two-thirds of a pound per day for twenty-one days on the Rotation Diet.* Some women, especially heavier women, will lose as much as a pound per day. Men may lose even more. But these are just the averages.

If you have a tendency to retain water, as many overweight persons do, you may lose as much as 2 or even 3 pounds a day during the first three days of the Rotation Diet. Many individuals lose two to three inches around the waist and buttocks in just three days, and, as you will see from the comments made by participants in our program (Chapter 3), you can be one or two dress or pants sizes smaller in three weeks or less. Thus, while the Rotation Diet is designed to help individuals who are significantly overweight, it is also the perfect diet for anyone who has struggled with the last 5 or 10 pounds that stand between them and their most desirable weight.

WHAT IS THE ROTATION DIET?

When you use the Rotation Diet you alternate your caloric intake over a three-week period in order to achieve a dramatic, quick weight loss without predisposing yourself to that frustrating rebound weight gain that tends to follow the use of every other low-calorie diet.

Women use a mixed diet consisting of a wide variety of foods and approximately 600 calories per day for three days, followed by 900 calories per day for four days, and then a week on 1200 calories per day. You then do the 600/900-calorie rotation once again.

Men use a mixed diet of approximately 1200 calories per day for three days, followed by 1500 calories per day for four days, followed by a week on 1800 calories per day. The 1200/1500 rotation is repeated once again.

Then, *you STOP dieting*. Weight loss has been so easy and so successful that you will want to continue if you have more weight to lose. But it is very important to the success of the Rotation Diet that you take at least a brief vacation from dieting. This brief vacation not only increases your motivation to succeed, *it helps guarantee that you do not regain any weight when you reach your goal weight*. I will explain why in just a moment.

After a week's or a month's vacation from dieting (it's up to you) you go on the Rotation Diet for another 10-, 15-, or 20-pound weight loss. Your motivation to succeed will never be greater. After all, how many times have you had to FORCE yourself to STOP dieting in order to ensure your success? With other diets, you soon begin to feel so deprived, and weight loss becomes so frustratingly slow, you just quit in disgust. Not so with the Rotation Diet. You will be itching to get going once again. The rotation is the key to your success. Even if you have up to 75 pounds to lose, the Rotation Diet is the surest way to get that weight off easily and quickly, *and keep it off.*

WILL YOU BE ABLE TO EAT LIKE A NORMAL HUMAN BEING AND NOT GAIN WEIGHT AFTER THE ROTATION DIET?

Yes! And that is the answer that we have all been searching for. For most of us, as hard as it might be to lose weight, it is still harder to keep weight off once lost than it is to get it off in the first place.

In order for you to appreciate the true significance of the Rotation Diet you need to understand why it is so easy to regain weight after a diet, especially quick-weight-loss diets other than the Rotation Diet. One of the reasons for that rebound weight gain is that when you go on a low-calorie diet (800 calories or less) for as few as three weeks, *your metabolic rate can slow down rather drastically.* This means that when you finish dieting you cannot eat anywhere near what you did before you began to diet without gaining weight. The process works in the following way.

The term *metabolic rate* refers to the speed with which your body burns calories. Your resting metabolic rate is the speed with which your body burns calories at rest, just doing the job of keeping itself alive—circulating blood, nourishing and rebuilding your body cells, thinking and problem solving, and so forth. Your total daily need for calories is determined primarily by your resting metabolic rate, plus the amount of physical activity you add to your life each day.

Although there is a great deal of variability, the average woman needs a total of between 1800 and 2000 calories per day in order to maintain her weight. The average man needs between 2400 and 2700. This total includes the number of calories it takes to maintain the body at rest, plus the amount needed for movement.

THE STARVATION RESPONSE

When a person goes on a low-calorie diet (especially a diet that ignores physical activity) a marvelous thing happens. It's called metabolic adaptation, or, simply, the "starvation response." As a result of millions of years of evolution in which the human race faced periodic famine, our bodies have developed an automatic, built-in ability to cut back on our need for calories if we cut back on our food intake. In some ways it's like turning down a thermostat to lower the heat in a house. Your body temperature falls, your heart rate slows down, other body functions slow down, all in an effort to conserve energy. This ability to slow down is very important in case we have to face a famine, as many hundreds of millions of people in the world still do each year.

However, the body's ability to slow down and cut back on its metabolic needs is not very helpful for an overweight person trying to maintain a weight loss after a low-calorie diet. Our research, and that of many others, shows that after a low-calorie diet, if you eat any more than 60 percent of what you used to eat before you began the diet, *you will start to gain weight*.

This will have a great deal more meaning for you if you think of what it takes to stay alive for an hour, just sitting still. The average nondieting woman might need 60 or so calories; the man, about 80. But after a low-calorie diet, the woman may only need 35 or 40; the man, 45 or 50. And even the caloric cost of activity will have been reduced. Before a diet, you normally burn up in the vicinity of 100 calories per mile of walking. After a diet, you may burn up only 60 calories per mile. So, if you are a victim of the starvation response and have reduced your metabolic rate through unwise dieting, you can't even get the normal weight-management benefits of exercise.

If you have tried a low-calorie diet plan for as long as three weeks you will now understand one reason why it was so easy to gain weight when you finished. And, since your body didn't need as many calories, you will also understand why it may have become more difficult for you to lose weight after you had regained it following a low-calorie diet.

The main point of all of this is that you should not do anything to lower your metabolic rate while dieting. In fact, you should be doing every healthy thing you can to increase your metabolic rate. The higher your metabolic rate, the better off you are, because that means you are burning up those calories that would otherwise turn to fat.

And now for the good news! REALLY good news.

The Rotation Diet does not slow metabolic rates.

I know you are going to be happy with the speed of weight loss on the Rotation Diet. But you are going to be even happier when you discover that the Rotation Diet will not predispose you to that rebound weight gain you may have experienced after using other fast-weight-loss plans, whenever you have tried to stabilize your weight.

Research using the Rotation Diet with participants in the Vanderbilt Weight Management Program shows that, in spite of a significantly increased rate of weight loss compared with the best non-rotation, strict 1200-calorie diet plan we had been able to devise, *there is no reduction in metabolic rate*. In fact, most participants using the Rotation Diet show an *increase* in metabolic rate. This means that instead of training their bodies to get along on less food while they are dieting, they are *increasing* their ability to eat after the diet without regaining weight.

The Rotation Diet short-circuits the starvation response for several reasons. First, you use a mixed diet containing a wide variety of foods (high-protein diets that cut out carbohydrates, such as bread, potatoes, fruits, and vegetables, are more likely to slow metabolic rate). Second, you don't stay on a caloric intake below 1200 calories for more than a week. And, third, if you are a sedentary person, you get more active.

Your final objective is, of course, to be able to eat like a normal healthy person without gaining weight. As part of the Rotation Diet maintenance plan, I will show you which foods and which exercises can increase your metabolic rate. Most people, with a wise choice of foods, can eat a good 20 percent more calories per day than they are presently eating and not gain weight!

HERE'S WHAT THIS BOOK CONTAINS

In the next two chapters I am going to tell you how the Rotation Diet came into being. First I'll tell you how I, personally, lost 75 pounds over twenty-two years ago, cured my hypertension, and

helped prevent a recurrence of the heart attack that started me on
the road to creating the program I am going to describe in this
book. Then I want to tell you about the research that demonstrat-
ed how effective the Rotation Diet could be in helping you to
achieve your own personal goals.

In Chapters 4 and 5 I will explain what you will need to do
to be as successful as the participants in the Vanderbilt Weight
Management Program when you use the Rotation Diet. I want to
tell you exactly what we tell them when they meet with us for
weekly supervision and guidance. Successful weight loss requires that you anticipate events, pressures, and temptations that
might interfere with your resolve to follow the Rotation Diet. If
you follow my advice I think you will be prepared for anything
and everything and end up having the most successful weight-
management experience of your life.

Then we get down to the nitty-gritty. In Chapters 6 and 7
I'll lay out the Rotation Diet and the exercise plan that can give
you that average of two-thirds of a pound of weight loss per day,
without increasing the likelihood of gaining weight in the future.

Chapter 8 will show you how to maintain your weight loss
as you take a vacation from dieting. In Chapters 9 through 11 I
will continue with a section on how to achieve weight-management
mastery. If you are overly fond of those rich foods we generally
call "junk food" (candy, desserts, high-fat snack foods), I'd like
to show you how to manage junk food in your diet, since there is
no way in the world that you are going to succeed in giving up
for life every single thing you like best. And, if you have been
overly hard on yourself, kicking yourself because of your past
inability to control your weight, you may have been feeding
yourself a lot of "mental junk food." I'd like to show you how
to deal with the garbage in the mental part of your diet, as well,
so that you, too, can become a weight-management champion.
You *can* manage your weight successfully.

Finally, just to keep your menus interesting and to illustrate
how well you can eat on a healthful weight-reducing and weight-
maintenance diet, I include in Chapter 12 a list of alternate
menus and recipes for the Rotation Diet that were designed by
our nutrition consultant, Ms. Rachel Willis.

SPECIAL HEALTH BENEFITS OF THE ROTATION DIET

The Rotation Diet will not only lead to rapid weight loss. It has many other significant health benefits.

On the average, there is a 10 percent reduction in serum cholesterol levels, and a 15 percent reduction in circulating triglycerides, even in persons whose cholesterol and triglyceride levels are not abnormally high to begin with. Of course, the more elevated these levels, the more benefit you can expect. (A high cholesterol level is a significant factor in cardiovascular disease, and high triglycerides have also been implicated.) Fasting glucose levels* tend to return to normal, if high, so that if your doctor has said that you have "high blood sugar," there is every likelihood that it will normalize, and stay normal, if you follow my maintenance suggestions. And, by the way, we have not seen a single case of low fasting blood sugar in persons using the Rotation Diet.

You will be interested in knowing that about 50 percent of all persons with mild essential hypertension will eliminate their need for medication with the loss of only about 10 percent of their body weight. Thus, you don't even have to reach ideal weight before you can obtain significant health benefits from the Rotation Diet.

A final word of advice before you begin. One of the first rules of good practice in the health field requires that my advice does not hurt anyone. We have a *perfect* record in the Vanderbilt Weight Management Program and I want it to stay that way. While the Rotation Diet can be used in reasonable comfort by persons in good health, no one should undertake this or any other fast-weight-loss program without consulting with his or her physician. The 600/900-calorie week in the Rotation Diet is not appropriate for diabetics. (If you are diabetic, the 1200-calorie plan is appropriate, and can be repeated indefinitely. Discuss it with your doctor.) If you are on any blood pressure medication,

---

*All blood chemistry work must be done after a twelve-hour fast, that is, first thing in the morning before breakfast, in order to be accurate and not reflect nutrients that are being absorbed into the bloodstream after a meal. This is standard medical practice.

including a diuretic, your need for medication may be reduced *or entirely eliminated in just a few weeks*. That's a fantastic health benefit of the Rotation Diet. However, your medication must be monitored during a diet. *Do not make any changes in your medication without your doctor's supervision*.

There are certain other important limitations in the use of the Rotation Diet in addition to the ones mentioned. The diet is not appropriate for children and adolescents, although if you show it to your doctor or nutritionist, especially the menus for Week 2 for both men and women, he or she will be able to suggest additions that will be suitable for your children. Some of these additions are mentioned later in the text. The diet is not suitable for pregnant women and nursing mothers, nor for people who are intensely active already—for example, persons who run several miles a day. In my opinion, active men and women should not cut more than 500 calories a day below their maintenance levels in order to lose weight and still maintain their health and energy levels.

Remember that this diet is meant to make you feel good, so if the addition of the *free vegetables* and *safe fruit* that I suggest in Chapter 6 during the 600-calorie rotation should not happen to be enough food to keep you energetic and in good spirits, do not hesitate to go up to 900 calories, or even to 1200. (Men on the 1200 rotation should go up to 1500 or 1800 calories.) Maintaining good health, mental and physical, during a diet is much more important than setting a weight-loss record.

Since this is a new diet, your doctor may not be aware of its details. The diet has been carefully designed with the Recommended Dietary Allowances of known vitamins and minerals in mind. One of our primary goals was to select foods that would maintain electrolyte balance (the correct ratio of potassium, for example, to other minerals) over the entire period in which you would use the Rotation Diet. In this, we have been entirely successful. Because many health professionals are concerned over the effects of any fast-weight-loss program, free copies of the daily plans, together with a summary report of the medical tests, which show beneficial changes in serum cholesterol, triglycerides, and fasting glucose without any harmful changes in electrolyte balance, will be sent to all physicians and other health professionals who write, on their letterheads, to the Vanderbilt Weight Management Program, 134 Wesley Hall, Vanderbilt University, Nashville, TN 37240.

2

How the Rotation Diet Came into Being: A Personal Success Story

Twenty-two years ago I weighed 75 pounds more than I do today. The way I lost that weight and kept it off for all these years forms the personal basis for the Rotation Diet. Perhaps because I really know from my own experience what it's like to be severely overweight and to have finally won my own battle, I have been able to inspire and help other individuals who have joined the Vanderbilt Weight Management Program be more successful than they would otherwise have been. I'm proud of what I have accomplished and I think you can do just as well, so, I'd like to tell you something about myself and how I did it.

I was one of those fat kids who had no memory of ever being thin. Instead, I have memories such as not being able to run fast enough to keep up with my playmates, being chosen last for all games that required physical movement, and being so fat by the age of four or five years that I couldn't even bend over in my snowsuit to make snowballs and enter into the snowball fights that filled the winter afternoons with excitement for children in the upper New York State city where I grew up. I found some small consolation in comparing myself with another

9

"little" fat boy. I used to keep repeating to myself, "I'm not the fattest boy in the class. Albert Rosenberg [that's not his real name] is fatter than I am." Perhaps poor Albert was consoling himself in a similar way, using me for comparison.

By the time I was twelve years old I was 50 pounds overweight. My parents became so concerned that they took me to the pediatrician for a visit that I will never forget. The doctor measured my body frame and, in my mind's eye, I can see him clearly this very moment, standing before me, running his finger along the diagonal of a chart, reaching the corner, looking down at me, emitting a surprised little chuckle, and saying, "You aren't even on the chart!"

I have fond memories of my childhood doctor even though I did not lose weight as a result of any of his efforts. I always had the feeling that he was trying to help me. After the appropriate tests, he determined that I was low in thyroid and had a slow metabolic rate. He placed me on thyroid medication and gradually increased the dosage up to 4 grains as I gradually upped my consumption of potato salad. He told my parents that they should encourage me to restrict my food intake, which they always did, but only after reminding me of the starving kids in Armenia (my parents were lucky enough to have left Russia at the turn of the century). I paid more heed to the needs of the starving kids in Armenia while I was eating than to my parents' admonitions to restrain myself, which always seemed to follow after I had finished. In the end, I began to have heart palpitations, the thyroid medication had to be discontinued, and my parents gave up on their efforts to control my eating.

By the time I reached thirty-five I was 75 pounds overweight and hypertensive. I remember the day that I had to lie down on a couch for an hour in order to bring my blood pressure down to 140/90 so that the examining physician would OK me for an insurance policy to cover the new house I had just purchased on moving to Nashville. And I certainly know the effort that is involved in lugging an extra 75 pounds of fat around! I would get out of breath just going across the street from my office and walking up one flight of stairs to the library. I remember putting off library visits until I had several tasks to do because of the effort involved in getting there and going up and down in the stacks.

My weight, inactivity, and genetic predisposition also blessed me with varicose veins by the time I was twelve. At that early age, I had my first attack of thrombophlebitis, which led to the injection treatment that was popular forty-five years ago and which resulted in permanent injury and disfigurement to one of my legs. Every two or three years I would suffer another attack, at times requiring me to spend as long as a month in bed, and two months more on crutches. Unfortunately, no physician was able to prescribe the treatment that finally ended this plague of inflammations and clotting in both of my legs—I had to discover it for myself at the age of fifty. Because so many people suffer from similar problems with their veins, I'll have more to say about this problem later.

Of course I tried many diets during these years. I tried grapefruit diets and egg diets. I tried fasting and even devised my own version of a powdered, high-protein diet. I would stuff gigantic capsules with gelatin, and swallow a package worth of capsules with two glasses of water for breakfast, and another package worth of capsules for lunch, with yet another two glasses of water. (You can imagine what I did for the rest of the day.) I could lose weight as fast as anyone. And put it back just as fast.

It finally happened while I was playing a game of ping-pong outside my office in the hallway of the Psychology Department, where we had set up a makeshift table. I began to get dizzy and nauseated, I broke out in a cold sweat, I could not catch my breath, and my knees began to quiver. Somehow I made it back to the chair in my office, but I did not want to face it: I was having a heart attack. I did not want to face it even though I had been having chest pains periodically for several years. I did not want to face it even though one time I had actually been knocked off my feet by the pain and unable to lift my arm.

I gradually returned to near normal in about forty-five minutes. I called my wife first, to tell her what had happened and to assure her that I felt all right but that I was about to get to a doctor. The cardiograms did indeed suggest that I had had a heart attack, and I am forever grateful to Dr. Ed Tarpley for the treatment he prescribed. It was 1963, just before the time when physicians began to do coronary bypass operations, so I was spared that operation, and my doctor tended to use medications as a last resort. Ed said simply, "You've got to lose that weight. I don't care what diet you use as long as it's a healthy one, but you *have got* to get active. That is the only way you will keep the weight off and possibly prevent another occurrence."

The clearest thing in my memory of the days that followed is the recurring thought that I wanted to stay alive as my children grew up. My daughter was eight and my son ten. And it was no time to leave my wife—our love and friendship have always been very special and then, as always, we had so much to look forward to together. Would I finally find a way to take the weight off in spite of all of my past failures? Would I be able to keep it off? I had no successful past behavior to guide me since there never was a time in my life when I had been thin. And could I find an activity that wouldn't hurt my legs and put me in bed with thrombophlebitis every other year? At that time, too much walking or the slightest bruise could do it. I knew no active games. I didn't even know what the inside of a gym might look like, and I certainly was not going to get inside one and undress so that everyone could see how fat and ugly I was.

Back in 1963 I did not know as much about the design of a diet for weight loss as I do now. (I was researching other areas of psychology having to do with the effects of anxiety on learning. The Vanderbilt Weight Management Program did not come into existence until 1976.) I did know one thing at that time, however, and that was—*something had to change!* You can't eat fatty foods, eat a lot of sweets, and consume large quantities of alcohol and lose weight easily.

So, I cut them all out. *ALL.* For periods of three weeks I was absolutely perfect. Then I would *stop* dieting and return to a normal eating pattern, which included those things we all seem to prefer in our diets. I never regained any of the weight I had lost. Without my realizing it, the principles that would form the basis of the Rotation Diet twenty-two years later were born.

What exactly was I doing and what had I learned? Here are a few of the main things:

First, I was following a quick-weight-loss plan that resulted in 15 to 20 pounds of weight loss each time I dieted.

Second, I never planned to diet more than three weeks at a time.

Third, I gradually increased my activity level, playing tennis every day (you will find an activity of your choice).

Fourth, by being active, and not dieting for more than three weeks at a time, I evidently did not lower my metabolic rate, nor did I increase the fat storage ability that seems to follow prolonged use of a low-calorie diet, *because I never regained any weight after each period of weight loss.*

Fifth, before going on each weight-loss rotation, I would get really motivated to be perfect, knowing that 15 to 20 pounds was about to come off and that I intended to stop after three weeks. (I must admit that I once continued to diet for four weeks because I found it very hard to stop at three when I was being so successful in losing weight.)

I learned much, much more about successful weight loss as I began to implement my plan. The insights I gained made it relatively easy—much easier than I ever expected. Many things occurred to help me lose 75 pounds in a little over a year that I did not actually plan or anticipate. I will tell you all about these things later in the book as I go along, showing step by step how I and other successful people actually implement the Rotation Diet. What I learned by chance, and trial and error, you can do intentionally.

As I write these introductory words, I am celebrating my fifty-seventh birthday. I can report that my blood pressure hovers right around 120/80, I have kept that 75 pounds off for twenty-two years, I was even able to quit smoking and keep the weight off, I have never had another heart attack (for which I also thank the good Lord), I love to get on the treadmill and watch that steady heartbeat on the polygraph as I approach maximum exertion, and I have not spent a single day in bed with either an inflammation or a blood clot in my legs after discovering what it takes to prevent their occurrence.

And I'm very, very glad to have stayed around, alive and healthy, to keep company with my wife and family, because as I reread and edit what I have written, I am looking forward to a special occasion. Tonight (October 19, 1985) the whole family will be together to celebrate my wife's fiftieth anniversary as a pianist when she performs Ravel's Piano Concerto in G Major with the Nashville Symphony Orchestra.

So mine has been a rewarding story. Now my hope is that what I have to say will be of help to you and add to the pleasure of your life.

3

How the Rotation Diet Came into Being: The Research

In spite of my own success with a quick-weight-loss program twenty-two years ago, I began our formal experiments on a quick-weight-loss diet in the Vanderbilt Weight Management Program with a number of misgivings.

First and foremost among my reasons for being reluctant to experiment with a quick-loss plan was that such plans have not been in accord with generally accepted practice in medicine and nutrition. I have always wanted to advise overweight persons to use an approach to weight loss that was as safe as a weight-loss program could possibly be, for everyone. Finally, after many years, I simply had to face reality. Although we had achieved outstanding success in the Vanderbilt Weight Management Program in comparison with other weight-loss programs, by following standard practice in our dietary recommendations we were not helping a majority of persons reach desirable weight.

Second, and I feel sure you will appreciate this if you are an overweight person, I wanted to be sure that, once you had lost the weight you wanted to lose, you would not have done anything to yourself through unwise dieting that would make it especially easy to regain that weight. Before we developed the Rotation Diet, the evidence against the long-term use of a low-calorie diet was quite clear. You might lose weight quickly, but, in part because of the slowdown in your metabolic rate (the starvation response), you would be unable to eat more than a fraction of your former intake without regaining your weight.

Third, I was sensitive to the desire on the part of overweight persons to get their weight off "as of yesterday." At least at the outset, most overweight persons don't want to consider losing their weight as I did, in blocks of 15 to 20 pounds at a time, with a "time-out" period between their periods of caloric restriction. No matter how much you have to lose, if you are like most overweight persons, you are likely to want to take it all off in one massive, prolonged assault. Although I always told our participants in the Vanderbilt Program about my own methods, I would advise them to follow a moderate diet (1200 calories per day for women, 1800 for men), and, in weekly counseling sessions, all of the group leaders in the Vanderbilt Program would attempt to help our participants stick with their diets for anywhere from ten to twenty weeks.

In other words, I was (and am) concerned with safety and long-term maintenance. Although in the past my colleagues and I thought it best to go along with everyone's initial desire to stick with a single prolonged attempt to lose every single pound of excess weight in one fell swoop, no matter how much they had to lose or how long it took, we no longer think that this is the best way to go about it.

It's not that the results with our old approach were turning out badly in the long run for persons with a modest amount of weight to lose. In comparison with the weight-loss and *weight-maintenance* records of most weight-control programs, we were doing very well. But, we were not at all as successful with this old, moderate approach as we and our participants would have liked.

Let me give you a brief summary.

PAST RESULTS: A REPORT ON THE OLD VANDERBILT PROGRAM

On the good side, 32.5 percent of all participants in the old (pre-Rotation Diet) Vanderbilt Program are in the desirable weight range as long as three years after their participation.

Twenty percent of the persons who had 40 pounds or more to lose did lose that much weight, and are keeping it off. Looking at our group averages, 85 percent of the weight that was lost during the program is being kept off. Compared with any other results of which we are aware, these achievements are outstanding.

We were, and, of course, still are, especially pleased with these weight-maintenance results. When we look at the follow-up questionnaires to determine why we have been so successful in maintenance, we see that persons who have been through the Vanderbilt Weight Management Program tend to put the sound nutritional principles they learn in the program *and* an increase in their daily activity *together* in their permanent programs for weight management. I am going to take special pains to show you how to be as successful in maintenance as they are.

On the bad side, however, when we looked at the weight-loss records of thousands of persons (in our old program as well as reports in the literature for programs like it), we saw that the average weight loss on any moderate weight-reducing diet recommended for women is only about 1 pound to 1½ pounds per week. The average weight loss for programs all around the United States lasting ten weeks is only about 10 pounds! In intensive (and expensive) programs lasting twenty or more weeks, for persons who are 50 to 125 pounds overweight, the average loss is 30 pounds. This is simply not good enough.

IT IS NOW MY OPINION THAT NO SLOW, MODERATE AP-PROACH TO WEIGHT REDUCTION WILL EVER WORK FOR THE MAJOR-ITY OF OVERWEIGHT PERSONS. This is especially true for women, who lose weight so much more slowly than men.

The problem is that most persons find it difficult, if not impossible, to follow the slow, moderate approach for very long. There are too many choices to make, we are surrounded by tempting high-calorie foods, and our family and outside social lives continually expose us to temptations that are hard to resist for more than a short period of time. Most of us can be "pretty good" for short periods, but in a matter of weeks, say even three or four, we begin to make those tiny deviations, followed by larger deviations, that bring our weight losses to a virtual standstill.

All of this means that the true focus of our past success, and of all programs that use moderate approaches, has been, and will continue to be, with a small percentage of persons who do not have very much weight to lose. Ten pounds—good. Twenty or twenty-five pounds—still pretty good. But even in these instances, with relatively small amounts of weight to lose, only a few can actually expect to make it all the way into the desirable weight range if they use a slow, moderate approach to weight loss.

So, although we are proud of our past success in helping participants keep off whatever weight they did lose, with that 85 percent weight-maintenance figure, as we looked at our less-than-perfect results we realized that *we had to keep prodding ourselves to find a way to help everyone lose ALL the weight they need to lose IN THE FIRST PLACE.* Then we could put our existing expertise to work in maintenance.

Considerations such as these kept me looking for ways to help people lose *more* weight and lose it *faster,* so that they would be inclined to remain motivated for whatever period it would take to be perfectly successful.

THE ROTATION DIET IS BORN

As I pondered different approaches to increasing the rate and total amount of weight our participants would lose, I kept returning to the method I had used myself twenty-two years ago—quick losses for three-week periods, and then a "time-out." My daily activity kept me from regaining weight. Then, when the spirit moved me, another rotation. It's true that "my way" of losing weight did not follow the guidelines that are part of standard practice in nutrition and "my way" was not what we had been encouraging our participants in the Vanderbilt Weight Management Program to follow, but I had lost over 75 pounds and kept them off for twenty-two years. How can you argue with such results? Had "my way" hurt me? On the contrary, I had been more successful than all but a handful of the persons I had been trying to help with "standard practice," and I am in excellent health.

What about my metabolic rate? It had been so low as a child that the pediatrician had me on 4 grains of thyroid medication. Now, however, my metabolic rate is actually about 15 percent higher than the average man of my age. I eat almost 3000 calories per day, which is about 15 percent more than the average man of fifty-seven years. And I don't gain weight. Whatever I did to lose weight, and whatever I am doing to keep it off, have not interfered with my metabolism. Instead, I am healthier than ever before, and my body has responded to my present healthy diet and active life-style by actually *increasing*, rather than decreasing, its daily need for food. At the personal level, I certainly know the secret of weight loss and weight maintenance. So I kept asking myself, "If my way of rotating my diet worked so well for me, why don't I break down and at least give it a shot? Why don't I at least try to adapt it for everyone who wants to try it?"

My major fear was that the beneficial results that I had experienced would not occur for everyone. However, many respected professionals all over the country were coming to the same realization as I: traditional dietary means, even when combined with the best that behavioral psychology had to offer, were not getting very much weight off the people who needed to lose more than 10 or 15 pounds. Many of these professional health workers were beginning to experiment with very-low-calorie diets, including powdered formula diets of as low as 400 to 600 calories a day for periods of up to two months, in an effort to find more effective weight-loss strategies. I did not want to use such diets because of the possibly serious metabolic consequences. (They can also have serious effects on cardiac function and require constant medical supervision.) And I have personally seen the rapid gain in weight that almost invariably follows the use of such diets.

Several things occurred that finally changed my mind about trying to design a quick-weight-loss diet.

First, with respect to the data on changes in metabolic rate that take place when a person begins to diet, it seems that little if any reduction occurs for several days. In fact, when some people start a diet, they seem to get excited. They experience a sort of "high" that might elevate the metabolic rate to a small extent temporarily.

Second, we and other researchers around the country had obtained evidence showing that, when a sedentary person increases physical activity, metabolic rates do not decrease, and may even increase, during moderate caloric restriction. Would activity also work to prevent the decrease if the diet were more severe?

Third, we were halfway through one of our ten-week programs during the fall/winter of 1984/85 when four of the eighteen women in one of my groups became dissatisfied with their rate of weight loss on our usual 1200-calorie diet. They were doing fine with their physical activity but they were having trouble making choices from the wide variety of foods we recommended and they were finding it difficult to maintain their motivation to continue to avoid the desserts and alcoholic beverages that have to be avoided, *if a person wants to lose weight quickly.*

So, I laid out my plan to rotate a quick-weight-loss diet with a period of rest, then start the quick loss again, similar to what I had done many years before. The women were extremely eager to try it. We would monitor their metabolic rates on a weekly basis, to determine whether or not a dramatic, but temporary, decrease in calories would lower their metabolic rates, which until that time had not suffered any decline.

The results caused a great deal of excitement. Although weight loss speeded up significantly, we could detect no decrease in metabolic rate. Morale skyrocketed and their motivation to continue with their weight-loss program was restored. These results encouraged me to plan a much larger trial in the spring and summer of 1985.

We recruited twenty women who wanted to participate in a test of the Rotation Diet right from the start of their weight-loss efforts. They began with three days on a 600-calorie diet, upped it to 900 for four days, then increased to 1200 for a week. Then they repeated the 600/900 rotation. Physical activity (walking or its equivalent in terms of energy expenditure) was gradually increased, with a goal of fifteen minutes per day the first week, up to forty-five minutes per day during the third week. We also set a target of a minimum of five days per week for activity, with six or seven preferred, provided it felt good! We obtained pre-program baseline resting metabolic rates and then we monitored these rates on a weekly basis. We also obtained answers to a set of questions that measured the ease of sticking with the plan and satisfaction with progress. Of course, we were eager to compare the speed of weight loss with the 1- to 1½-pound weekly loss that is usually obtained with the 1200-calorie diets.

RESULTS WITH THE FIRST CLINICAL TRIAL USING THE ROTATION DIET

In a nutshell, the results were fantastic. The average weight loss was 12.5 pounds in twenty-one days. That's about two-thirds of a pound a day. The heaviest women lost as much as a pound a day. There was no reduction in resting metabolic rate; in fact, there was a small (but statistically insignificant) metabolic increase. Ninety percent of the women said they preferred the Rotation Diet to the slower, more moderate diets they had tried in the past, and I had a great deal of difficulty persuading them to take that vacation from dieting (for at least one week) that is an essential part of the plan.

SOME PERSONAL REACTIONS TO THE ROTATION DIET

To formally monitor reactions to the diet each week, we had participants fill out a questionnaire. Here are some of the comments that are in our written records:

"It's so clear. You can't make a mistake!"

"It works!"

"The 600/900 is easy to stay on—fewer choices, fewer temptations."

"Very happy with this diet plan. Can't think of anything bad to say about it."

"The best thing about this diet is that I feel thinner (and better)."

"I am really having a good time on my walks. When I've lost weight before I've found it difficult to lose in my hips and thighs, but because of the walking this is the first place I'm losing. I've already gone down one entire dress size, and two in pant size [after one rotation]. I love it."

"The best—plenty to eat and pleasant variety of foods [on the 1200 part of the rotation]."

"When I reach the 1200 calories per day I really feel rewarded for having been so good on the 600/900."

"I feel better and have more energy."

"It works, and I'm really building self-esteem."

"I see the results I started out to accomplish."

"The 600/900 part is even easier than I thought it could possibly be."

Obviously, with such outstanding results, we had to make the Rotation Diet a part of our regular weight-loss program for persons who do not have any physical condition that makes its use unwise.

NOW IT'S YOUR TURN!

And when you finish, I want you to write to me to tell me how well the Rotation Diet has worked for you. (Follow the instructions for writing given in Appendix B.) First, study the plan and put it into practice, exactly as I tell you, for those three weeks that can result in an average of two-thirds of a pound to a pound a day of weight loss. Then write to me because I want to find out if a significant number of overweight persons can lose weight with the help of a book like this, just as well as they can in our program. You see, the only way that I can be successful as a professional trying to help people lose weight is if *you* are successful! There is no way of finding that out unless you tell me.

If you write to me, I'll put you on my follow-up maintenance list. Then you will hear from me periodically to find out how you are doing. Being on our follow-up list will help you stay motivated until your new thin life-style becomes so rewarding you will never go back to being fat, and your responses will give us needed information on long-term success in dealing with overweight. So, it will be of great benefit to both of us if you write, and I am encouraging you to do so.

4

Gearing Up for
the Rotation Diet

Timing, planning, commitment. These are the keys to success. Let me explain what I mean.

I realize that there is no perfect time to start a diet, but some times are better than others. Don't pick a time to start the Rotation Diet when everything in your life will conspire to make you deviate from your plans. If you are a woman, you would have to be a masochist to begin Week 1 of the Rotation Diet, in which you will be adhering to a 600-calorie diet for three days, followed by a 900-calorie diet for four days, if that week coincides with a festive period such as a holiday, an anniversary, or some other celebration. Right before and right after a holiday is just fine, since this is the rotation in which you will approximate a pound a day of weight loss. Thus, the week after the Christmas holidays is a great time to use Week 1 of the Rotation Diet and take off 5 or more pounds, and some women use Week 1 right before Christmas to lose 5 pounds, since this promotes the relative freedom of a 1200-calorie diet during the holiday week itself. But you should never punish yourself by trying to exercise anything more than modest restraint *during* festive periods. It just creates tension that can, in the end, lead to greater overeating than if you had not tried to be so extreme in the first place.

So, survey the weeks ahead. The best time for your first rotation will be when you can see three upcoming weeks in which you can plan to follow the Rotation Diet without anticipating a whole array of circumstances likely to encourage failure. You want three weeks in which the temptations to deviate will be about as low as you can expect them to be, considering your life situation.

Then, you must make a decision to be absolutely perfect in following the Rotation Diet.

PERFECT?

That word frightens you, doesn't it? If you could be perfect when it came to your eating habits, you wouldn't need to go on a diet!

Your feelings indicate that you don't have confidence in your ability to get the job done. You can't even *imagine* yourself being successful, and if you can't imagine yourself being successful, how in the world will you ever be able to do it in reality? I suspect that you may have had too many failures in the past to trust yourself on any plan that calls, from the start, for perfection.

If you have feelings such as these, then, at this point, *I have more faith in you than you have in yourself!* And I think I can show you how to develop all the confidence that you will need to succeed.

I have faith in you and in the plan because the Rotation Diet is, first of all, so easy to follow. Second, the steps to mastery that I will show you in Chapters 9 through 11 will help you achieve perfection, or near-perfection, with just a little bit of practice and enough initial commitment to start. And when I speak of that two-thirds of a pound per day of weight loss that you can expect with the Rotation Diet, I include in the data even those who make it to *nearly* perfect, using a couple of insurance policies that I explain in Chapter 6. Finally, I also know from experience that persons who aim for perfection from the start end up doing the very best.

The reason I ask you to demand perfection of yourself, and to develop the frame of mind that keeps you striving for it, is that changing your weight is, in the beginning stages, one of the hardest things you may ever undertake in your life. It takes fantastic commitment. The secret of success lies partly in the attitude with which you approach the task, and partly in having a strategy that yields a payoff worthy of your efforts. Then, once you see and feel the payoff, weight-management difficulties will be reduced considerably and you will wonder why it seemed so hard at first.

After you see what the diet requires, as well as the exercise program (Chapters 6 and 7, respectively), *you must take about half an hour to sit down and plan how to be perfect*. In those two chapters I'll show you, in detail, how to make your plans.

Here is the way I put the issue to participants in my groups in the meeting before we begin the Rotation Diet:

Three weeks of perfection is not too long to ask from anyone who is serious about weight loss. Think about it—I am not asking you to start a diet and stick with it for an indefinite period. You are not going to force yourself to stick with it until any set amount of weight is lost. You are going to plan for a limited time—*three weeks*—and in these three weeks you will actually have one week that demands relatively little of you. Upping your calories to 1200 per day, after the 600/900 rotation, feels like a tremendous reward. If you feel any pressure to deviate during the 600/900 rotation, simply look ahead to the 1200-calorie week, and wait with anticipation. Follow my advice and the results will be superb. Is it worth it to you to lose an average of two-thirds of a pound a day over that twenty-one day period—maybe even a pound a day?

Okay—you are only human. Suppose something happens that is so overwhelming you cannot resist deviating from your plans. Never interpret this kind of event as ultimate defeat—you have only lost a skirmish. Aim for the best you can do, accept your humanness, and aim once again for perfection. You will get better at it—I'll show you how. If you have more than 15 or 20 pounds to lose, your second twenty-one-day rotation on the diet will be even better than the first.

After this preamble, I go on to tell my group participants in the Vanderbilt Program about some of my personal experiences.

I learned a great deal about attitude, commitment, and strategy when I set out to lose those 75 pounds twenty-two years ago. In view of my health, weight loss had finally become a very important goal. Weight loss has to be an important goal for you, too, because I cannot supply the initial motivation for you to begin—I can show you how to reach your goal quickly and easily, reinforcing your motivation to succeed, but you have to have enough motivation to put the whole plan into action.

As I thought about the kind of diet I would follow in my own efforts to lose weight, I realized that I would have to find a way to cut out *all* things that are considered ''dense-calorie'' foods if I didn't want to dilly-dally around and take forever. That is, cakes, pies, cookies, ice cream, candy, alcohol, fried foods—

in fact, everything that has fat or sugar as the primary source of calories had to go. I knew, from many past failures, that when I included such foods while trying to lose weight I could play around with the same 5 or 10 pounds forever, losing and gaining, losing and gaining, and I would never make permanent progress. I'm sure that this comes as no surprise to you!

But I also knew that I, like most other people who love best the very foods we have to give up in order to lose weight efficiently, could not ask myself to exercise perfect restraint forever. I needed a goal, it had to be attainable, and it had to be explicit.

So I asked myself how long I thought I could be perfect if I had a good diet and a good plan for sticking with it. There were three weeks left of the summer vacation before classes resumed at Vanderbilt, so I arbitrarily decided on three weeks. As for the diet, it was going to be plenty of fruits and vegetables, together with lean meat, fish, fowl, and low-fat cheeses (I don't care much for milk, except with chocolate cake, apple pie, cookies, and peanut butter and jelly sandwiches). I decided to go light on bread (something I would not do today) because I could not imagine myself eating bread in those days unless it was hidden under a slab of butter.

So I had a time limit and the principles on which to build my diet. Now the question was, "Will I be able to stick it out for the full three weeks?"

My family was a great help and I'll talk more about how they came to help me when I discuss the steps you need to take to prepare your environment and other people for success. There is no way that I could have been as successful as I have been without the complete support I received, and continue to receive, from my wife and children.

With my family strongly behind me, my major fear was how to deal with lunches out each day, five days a week, in restaurants near my office, and the once- or twice-a-week dinner out or other social situation that had so often led me astray in my previous efforts to lose weight.

My fears were soon dispelled in a way that I did not fully appreciate until I reflected on it some years later. We were out to dinner with some good friends at a steak house, where I started off with a shrimp cocktail, followed by steak and a salad. My companions remarked on my "control"—I had passed on the hot bread and butter, and had been sipping my glass of ice water as they enjoyed their cocktails. They asked me what diet I was using and it just popped out, without much planning, because I had just noticed that everything I had been eating began with the letter "s"—"It's my own diet. I call it the 4S-Diet, and it's unlimited indulgence in shrimp, steak, salad, and sex."

The name of my diet got a few laughs and, since everyone began to notice that I was losing weight so quickly, I began to respond to all questions about what diet I was on with, "The 4S-Diet." My description was always worth a chuckle or two, but I soon discovered that it was worth much, much more than a little laugh. It disarmed potential temptors and temptresses. *No one, ever, at any party, dinner, or other social engagement, ever pushed me to deviate from my diet once I made my statement*. So I found it easy to adhere to it, sticking, in reality, not just to the four S's, but to a wide variety of fruits, vegetables, lean meats, fish, and fowl.

I had started my three weeks of dieting with commitment, and each time I announced and described the diet to someone else, that commitment grew. No matter what the temptation, I communicated unequivocally in all situations that I meant it when I said I was on a diet. Furthermore, talking about it in public whenever the occasion arose, as it almost always did on social occasions because so many people are interested in diets, was especially reinforcing. I lost between 15 and 20 pounds each time I went on my three-week diet. That amount of weight loss was always dramatic. All together—the quick loss, the humorous name for my diet, the public statement, and the reactions, with no one even unconsciously making any effort to sabotage my endeavor—all of these factors combined for a snowball effect. It was almost more fun to be on the diet and get these reactions and reinforcements than it was to be off it.

The Vanderbilt Weight Management Program did not come into being until thirteen years after I had lost all of my weight. It was only then, when I began to analyze the reasons for my success in sticking with a diet and to compare them with the reasons so many others seem to fail, that I appreciated the value of each component that I had in part planned and in part chanced upon. Let me summarize:

A reachable, time-limited goal—three weeks of dieting, and then a vacation.

A very reinforcing rate of weight loss

A bit of humor (which always helps to keep your spirits up while working on a difficult task)

An unequivocal public statement, made in such a way that it reflected my complete commitment and received complete respect

Public appreciation and reinforcement

Self-reinforcement (''bragging'' about my diet, which is something you can start doing with the Rotation Diet; a bit of bragging will help you, too)

The support of my family

In the next chapter I will show you some specific ways to apply all of my own personal experience, together with all the professional experience I have gained in helping others, to your own weight-management efforts.

5

Getting Started
on the Right Foot

In the previous chapter I gave you some general principles that will assure your success on the Rotation Diet. Now I want to give you three important specific suggestions.

First, take charge of your social environment. Make sure your family, friends, and co-workers know what you are about to do. If the people in your environment can have an impact on your behavior (and they usually can and do) you will do better with their complete cooperation.

Second, take charge of your physical environment. Make sure the physical aspects of your home and place of work will support your efforts in every way possible.

Third, make sure you have exactly the foods you plan to eat during the Rotation Diet already available when you start the diet, and plan your menus according to the directions I give you in the next chapter. If you plan to eat any meals in restaurants during the three weeks of the Rotation Diet, you will need to follow my special recommendations for dining out. I was able to eat lunches in a restaurant five days a week, and go out to dinner occasionally, too, and still succeed. So can you.

SETTING UP YOUR WORLD
TO SUPPORT SUCCESS

I don't think I could possibly have succeeded as easily as I did in losing weight and keeping it off without getting complete support from my family and setting up my daily schedule to facilitate weight loss.

I announced my intentions to my wife and requested that, for three weeks, we not bring any foods into the house that would tempt me to eat something that was not on my plan. After all, it was only for three weeks. Everyone wanted me to succeed, so I had no problem doing this. We brought no ice cream into the house during this period, and we baked no cheesecakes, both of which happen to be among my favorite high-calorie foods.

You may wonder why I decided to remove temptation completely, right from day one, rather than learn to deal with my appetites and change my eating habits gradually. The answer is quite simple: I wanted to lose weight quickly. I had no time to wait while I learned which behavior-change strategies would work and which would not when it came to resisting temptation. That could wait for the periods when I experimented with *maintenance,* not weight loss. Besides, I really like ice cream and cheesecake. There was no way in the world I could fool myself into disliking my favorite foods, keep them around the house for the entire period in which I was going to be losing weight, and not end up eating them.

Fortunately, I discovered as I went through my rotation diet that I didn't need to change my attitudes about food—I love to cook and I love to eat a wide variety of foods that include some dishes that nutritional ''purists'' would do away with entirely. I discovered a strategy that lets me live with and enjoy all of these foods once again in amounts that bear no danger for my weight, and I plan to show you how I and other successful participants from the Vanderbilt Weight Management Program do it.

However, when it comes to implementing the very best strategy for weight loss—*removing all temptation temporarily from your home*—you, unfortunately, may not find that your family is as cooperative as mine, especially if you are a woman! Even for that brief three-week period that I am suggesting, you may meet with almost insurmountable resistance. You are likely to hear, ''Why do we have to go on a diet because you are trying to lose weight?'' This response, generally received by women, makes me very angry. In fact, after working to help almost three thousand women in the Vanderbilt Weight Management Program lose weight, I can't express just how angry I am at my fellow males when it comes to helping the women they say they love to lose weight. In comparison with women, men with families usually have no problems when they announce they are ready to lose weight. Everyone rallies round, out goes the junk food, Mom makes low-calorie main dishes, and everyone falls in line to take care of things when Dad goes out to exercise. When Dad makes an unequivocal statement about what he wants, most families seem ready to cooperate.

In part because of the family cooperation that males receive, they find it much easier to lose weight. They also find it much easier to stay active after weight loss. But I can't find words to tell you how frustrated I am with the mates of the women in my groups. I am embarrassed and ashamed of male insensitivity to the problems that women face. Even today, when we are so much more likely to preach ''equality'' and cooperation in our marriages than was the case twenty-two years ago when I lost my weight, it still seems to be more talk than action. Men still get more support and encouragement for the decision to lose weight than women do. Husbands seem to expect their wives to maintain the status quo, and so do the children. You (woman, wife, and mother) are expected to keep all the tempting foods in the house and you will be made to feel like an ogre if you don't want to keep a daily dose of candy and cookies around for the children. You will be expected to continue to prepare all the high-fat and high-sugar dishes to which the family has been accustomed, continue to be not only a mom and wife, but possibly also a career woman, and certainly not inconvenience anyone with a change in your diet or physical activities because you would like to be healthier, happier, and more pleased with yourself.

Watch out, however, for something very subtle in your own attitudes about what you feed the family. As the saying goes, you may be caught ''between a rock and a hard place.'' You, like an amazing number of women, may not feel like a ''good mother'' or ''good wife'' unless you provide your family with junk food. You may obtain a great deal of satisfaction from the joy your family derives from eating these foods. As a woman, wife, and mother who cares for her family, you may not feel that you are showing that love, or that you are, yourself, fully loved or lovable, unless you see your brood relishing those high-fat and high-sugar foods that are not particularly good for anyone's health on a daily basis. You may be equating love and caring with the food you feed the family! Watch out! If you share any of the feelings I am talking about, you should stop and think—and realize that equating love and caring with the cookie jar does no one any good. You are not doing anyone a favor with a *daily* diet of junk food.

WEIGHT LOSS AND WEIGHT MAINTENANCE REQUIRE DIFFERENT STRATEGIES

Before going on with the recommendations for ensuring success while using the Rotation Diet for the next three weeks, I want to make some contrasts between what leads to the very best and most efficient weight loss and what I think works best for maintenance. Weight loss and weight maintenance are very different matters.

During each three weeks on the Rotation Diet, you aim for perfection, and the closer you get, the better you will do. After all, you can't lose two-thirds of a pound a day without sticking to the plan very closely. Removing temptation from your home environment and avoiding it elsewhere are the easiest ways to come close to perfection.

As for the long term, *it's balance and moderation, NOT striving for perfection,* that will ensure success in maintenance. Some of our successful participants call their approach to incorporating high-calorie foods into their diets "controlled bingeing"! They intentionally plan to include some every week. They avoid being overly restrained because they find that trying to be too perfect for too long can actually set them up for long-term failure. If you are at all like them, you, too, may have found that constant denial only increases your drive for dense-calorie foods. Then, the moment you indulge in a single bite, the floodgates open and you are overwhelmed by the appetite that has been building up. Thus, in maintenance, you control the appearance of temptations, having periodic indulgences that never let your drive to eat sweet and fatty foods build up to the point where you will overeat and put on weight.

In Chapters 9, 10, and 11, you will learn the strategies for self-mastery and environmental control that allow for "controlled bingeing" without regaining any weight after you have reached your goal. Just as ice cream and cheesecake are back in my present maintenance diet (together with a couple of beers after a nice jog in the park), your favorite high-calorie foods will return to your diet. But you will be in control, deciding just how many and how much of these foods you want to eat, and when.

So, to repeat, during the Rotation Diet you will find the task far easier if you remove temptations from your home environment. I hope you will be able to do this. If you are a woman, talk it over with your husband, and make plans for him and the rest of the family to have their ice cream, cookies, cakes, and candy as special treats away from home. It will be good for Dad to go out with the kids—they'll love him for it and it will give you a chance to go for a walk alone!

(If you are one of those persons who cannot, or who doesn't want to, remove temptations from your home, or who knows that temptations will be unavoidable in your social situation, read Chapters 9 through 11 before you begin. There I describe a strategy that yields a 95 percent success rate among participants in the Vanderbilt Program when they need special help in developing their resistance for the three weeks of the Rotation Diet.)

WHAT ABOUT EATING OUT?

I had lunches out, every day, five days a week, all during my periods of quick weight loss. Here's how.

I found a small grill near my office that would serve me one of three dishes that I had on my diet plan. The first was the dieter's special, a 6-ounce lean hamburger patty, with a selection of two side dishes from the following list: small dinner salad, sliced tomato and lettuce, cole slaw, cottage cheese, or sliced fruit. The second dish was "soup of the day," usually either vegetable, tomato, cream of mushroom, or split pea, which I would have with two small packages of crackers. The third was a large vegetable salad, which I would have with one tablespoon of dressing. For three weeks, I ate every single lunch at this restaurant. Thus I exposed myself to no special temptations. The waitresses at the grill, as well as the owner, got to know me very well and supported my diet plans. They greeted me with,

"What's it going to be today, Doc—salad, soup, or the hamburger?"

I have already explained how I used my "4S-Diet" label to ward off my "well-intentioned" friends who might tempt me to deviate on social occasions. If invited out to dinner at someone's home, I always let them know when I was in my "diet cycle." For me, it was skip the drinks, no dessert (other than fruit and a piece of cheese), don't pass the bread, and scrape off the sauce if my host had the audacity to prepare something that was especially rich for the main course.

I used similar strategies for eating out at restaurants. I always suggested that we go someplace where I would have no difficulty sticking with my diet. Selfish? Hell, no! That 15-pound loss was really worth it, and I had more at stake with that one meal out than anyone else in the crowd. For me, it was my life.

We never failed to find a place where everyone could be satisfied.

If you must eat out socially, think about your plan of action in advance, just as I did. Talk it over with your dinner companions and set up your support system. Just remember—most dieters fail on their diets because they are in conflict. They want to eat the foods they must temporarily deny themselves, so they find themselves "cooperating with circumstances" and setting themselves up for failure. You must make an unequivocal statement about your intentions, to yourself and to others, once you have made up your mind to follow the Rotation Diet. And the more you repeat the statement, publicly, as well as silently to yourself, the more you will reinforce your intentions and assure your success.

If you work outside the home, it's a good idea to think about how you will face the temptations that will occur during work breaks as well as at lunchtime. Your place of work will probably not offer a perfect environment for weight control. The cafeteria and snack machines will still have their fried foods and junk foods, even when they do offer healthful alternatives.

So what are you going to do?

Here's how I did it. I didn't want to be caught unprepared when I felt like a snack. To this day I carry bread and fruit to the office. I eat what I have brought for snacks, even if I join someone else. And, for lunch, if I eat out, my colleagues and I always go where we can choose healthful dishes. We also go where we are served, not where we must choose from a buffet. I do not like to submit myself to the temptations of a buffet—I find myself in conflict, fighting my desire to eat all of my money's worth and then some (I still remember the starving children in Armenia), knowing that if I do I will probably feel sleepy afterward, or uncomfortable when I go out for a jog or play tennis at the end of the day.

If you are a woman about to begin the Rotation Diet, during the week that you are on the 600/900-calorie phase you will do best if you carry your own lunch and avoid eating out. The lunches are easy to prepare and there is no problem preserving them until time to eat. When you are in the 1200-calorie week, there is more leeway for eating out. Men will have little trouble finding a way to eat out since they never drop below 1200 calories a day.

A FINAL WORD OF ADVICE

The Rotation Diet is the best quick-weight-loss plan that I know of—if you can be close to perfect, you can expect to average an enviable two-thirds of a pound of weight loss per day over the next three weeks. But I know the unexpected is to be expected. By that I mean, you may feel an almost irresistible urge to eat something not on the plan simply because someone puts it right in front of your nose and catches you off guard. A party occurs at work, for example. Or, you find yourself dying for a little something before going to bed, which is likely to happen to folks who are accustomed to one large, continuous meal from the time they get home from work until they go to sleep at night.

Of course, things such as I have just described happened to me while I was losing weight. Because I did not want to feel deprived, and I did not want to go to bed hungry, I decided I needed to have a "safe food" that I liked reasonably well and of which I could eat almost unlimited quantities without doing much damage to my weight-loss efforts.

However, choosing a "safe food" presented me with a problem. I just don't care much for the so-called "free foods" that anyone (you included) can always eat in unlimited quantities. (Free foods include lettuce, parsley, watercress, cucumbers, celery—I'll give you a complete list in the next chapter. I needed something that was more satisfying than the free foods, but still healthful and filling, while containing relatively few calories.

I decided that my safe food would be a fruit (and I now call it a *safe fruit*). Compared with other foods, fruit provides the most satisfaction in taste and bulk for the least amount of calories. And, in addition, I wanted something I liked so that it would be a reasonable substitution of foods that are much higher in calories.

I selected grapefruit as my safe fruit. A whole grapefruit has only about 110 calories. I carried one to the office in my briefcase and made a vow that I would have to eat that grapefruit instead of any high-calorie snack that happened my way. At least, I would say to myself that I had to eat it first, and then, if I wanted to, I could eat something else. But I never did. All the while that I peeled the grapefruit, I thought about how well I was losing weight, and how the high-calorie snack would slow me down. I would then break the grapefruit up into sections, and eat them, one at a time, as slowly as I could. If I was still hungry when I finished, I would drink a large glass of water.

I did the same at night at home whenever I felt hungry before going to bed. Sometimes I ate two grapefruits, peeled and sectioned. It is hard to be hungry after two whole grapefruits!

I don't want you to feel deprived, either, on the Rotation Diet, so I want you to choose a *safe fruit* just in case you, too, don't care very much for the free foods. I want you, too, to take a vow that your safe fruit is the only extra food you will eat while you are following the plan, no matter what temptations present themselves. In this way, you may end up losing only 10 pounds, rather than 15 or 20, during the next three weeks, but you will be prepared to resist the worst the world has to offer and you will not end up "blowing it all" and feeling frustrated.

I will give you a list of safe fruits in the next chapter, which describes the Rotation Diet. Choose one from the list. Have plenty at home and have some with you at all times. Your safe fruit will soon begin to act like a charm, protecting you from your old fat self, as well as from the temptations in your environment. In just two or three days, your friends will become accustomed to seeing you dip into your bag, purse, or briefcase for your healthful snack, and they will no longer encourage you to deviate. You, too, will be surprised at your own demonstration of willpower. Reaching for your safe fruit becomes a very simple thing to do—almost automatic, in fact. When you begin to feel a bit proud, even smug, over your ability to say "No, thanks" to temptation as you reach for your safe fruit, you can be sure that you are securely on your way.

And you can give any odds you like to anyone silly enough to bet against you that you will end up considerably thinner and stay that way.

6

The Rotation Diet
for Women and Men

I want to emphasize once again, before you begin the Rotation Diet, why you need to follow the suggestions I am making very closely.

The Rotation Diet, followed exactly as described in this chapter, does not lead to a reduction in your metabolic rate. I mean by this that you will need just as many calories to maintain yourself at a lower weight after you finish the diet and follow my instructions for maintenance as you did before you began the diet. Unlike other quick-weight-loss diets, the Rotation Diet does not make it easier for you to get fat all over again, after you stop dieting.

In this chapter I will lay out the complete dietary plan for women and men. *Do not start on the Rotation Diet until you have read Chapter 7, which describes the Rotation Diet activity program.* If you are interested in permanent weight control, you must implement the entire plan.

GENERAL INSTRUCTIONS

For Women

Women follow a rotation plan during Week 1 that includes approximately 600 calories a day for three days, followed by 900 calories a day for the next four days. In Week 2, you eat approximately 1200 calories a day for the entire week. In Week 3, you repeat the 600/900-calorie rotation. You can repeat the menus of Week 1 during Week 3, or, if you desire more variety, you can use the Alternate Menus for the Rotation Diet in Chapter 12.

It is very important for women to follow the Week 2 menus, which call for an increase in food intake to around 1200 calories. If you do not, you may reduce your metabolic rate. In addition, the increase feels like a feast and does wonders for your motivation. After what feels like a week of hardly being on a diet, you will be eager to get back on the 600/900-calorie rotation once again for another quick weight loss. Your weight loss in Week 2 will, of course, be less than in Weeks 1 and 3, but the increase in calories helps prevent regaining weight after you finish your diet. This protection is worth the temporary slowdown.

For Men

Men follow a rotation plan during Week 1 that includes approximately 1200 calories a day for three days, followed by 1500 calories a day for the next four days. In Week 2, you eat approximately 1800 calories a day for the entire week. In Week 3, you repeat the 1200/1500-calorie rotation. You can repeat the menus of Week 1 during Week 3, or, if you desire more variety, you can use the Alternate Menus for the Rotation Diet in Chapter 12.

It is very important for men to follow the Week 2 menus, which call for an increase in food intake to around 1800 calories. If you do not, you may reduce your metabolic rate. Eighteen hundred calories a day will hardly feel like a diet and the "time-out" it gives you will add to your motivation to return to the 1200/1500 rotation for another quick weight loss. Your weight loss in Week 2 will be less than in Weeks 1 and 3, but the increase in calories helps prevent regaining weight after you finish your diet. This protection is worth the temporary slowdown.

Expected Weight Loss

On the average, persons who follow the Rotation Diet exactly as printed will lose over 5 pounds the first week, around 2½ pounds the second week, and up to around 5 pounds again the third week. The heavier you are to begin with, the more you can expect to lose, up to an average of about a pound a day for the twenty-one days. And even though the calorie intake for men is higher, men will tend to lose faster than women. Men need more calories than women to maintain their initial weight and they burn more calories in physical activity because they are heavier.

PERMISSIBLE VARIATIONS ON THE ROTATION DIET

The Rotation Diet permits some variations that make it possible for persons who have trouble sticking with low-calorie diets to use it and still be very successful. I include these variations because some women may need to have a little more food than the basic 600/900-calorie rotation allows in order to avoid feeling empty at certain times of the day. The same goes for men who may find it difficult to stick exactly to 1200 calories. If you are such a person, you need to know what you can do without appreciable damage to your efforts. Other persons, such as nervous nibblers or persons who find themselves on a food expedition the moment they have nothing particularly demanding to do and begin to feel a little bored, also need to have something to fall back on as a snack that will not hurt the overall effectiveness of the diet.

Here are the permissible deviations that allow the diet to remain effective. These deviations include the use of *free vegetables* and a *safe fruit*. Together they constitute your insurance policy. Our research shows that women who include some of the permitted deviations may lose, on the average, only half a pound a day, but they still end up with a loss of 10½ pounds in twenty-one days. Be sure to follow these directions so that you can adhere to the plan for the full three weeks with the least damaging deviations, no matter what happens!

DIRECTIONS FOR USING FREE VEGETABLES

Certain foods have so few calories that you can eat them in unlimited quantities. They are called *free vegetables*. That is, because of their water and fiber content, relative to the number of calories they contain, you cannot eat enough of them to prevent yourself from losing weight, provided you follow my other suggestions exactly. Thus, whenever you see "unlimited free vegetables" on my menus, you can eat from the following list of vegetables until you feel satisfied (if you add salad dressing, use only my No-Cal Dressing, page 75, or a no-calorie commercial variety).

You are also permitted to add *free vegetables* to any meal and to nibble on them as snacks. Because they contain so many vitamins and minerals (plus fiber) in relation to their caloric content, you will be increasing the nutritional value of your diet tremendously if you do so. (*Free vegetables* have fewer than 10 calories per serving. If you are interested in more exact caloric values, see Appendix A.)

asparagus	endive	radish
celery	escarole	spinach
chicory	lettuce	watercress
Chinese cabbage	parsley	zucchini
cucumber		

DIRECTIONS FOR CHOOSING A SAFE FRUIT

The *free vegetables* just listed will help round out your meals so that you never have to feel hungry when you have finished the prescribed lunch or dinner. But if you are at all like me, free vegetables are not always satisfying—they don't have much flavor eaten alone, and, perhaps more important, they have so few calories that they don't give you any lift when you may really need one. That's why I think you should choose a *safe fruit* to fall back on whenever you feel hungry *between* meals or are tempted by some rich dessert. That's what I did twenty-two years ago when I decided that whenever I felt like a bedtime snack, or whenever I felt hungry between meals, I would peel and eat a whole grapefruit, *but only grapefruit and nothing else*, for the entire three weeks of my diet. By sticking with this vow I never failed to lose at least 15 pounds over any three-week period, and I never had to feel hungry!

Safe fruits do contain calories: from 40 calories for a small apple to 110 calories for a whole grapefruit. For this reason, they can give you a lift when you feel low on energy. The lift (and the bulk provided by the water and fiber) helps you stick with your diet until the next regular meal. The fruit sugar that they contain makes a safe fruit taste pretty good—not as good as your favorite high-calorie foods, perhaps, because safe fruits don't contain any fat, but good enough to get you by in a pinch. You must keep reminding yourself that every time you choose a safe fruit you are avoiding a choice of food that would prevent you from losing weight.

Choosing a *safe fruit* is very important from a psychological standpoint. It becomes symbolic of your weight-loss effort. You carry it with you to work and it's always available at home. Every time you get the urge to deviate from the Rotation Diet you reach for your safe fruit. Believe me, it's a charm! It's your absolute guarantee of success. Even if you have two or three servings a day during the 600/900-calorie rotations—a mid-morning snack, a mid-afternoon snack, a bedtime snack—you cannot add much more than 150 to 200 calories to your intake. Should you go further and add three whole grapefruit, which is considered to be six servings of fruit, you will add only 330 calories, and *YOU WILL STILL LOSE WEIGHT.* It may be only 8 or 10 pounds in three weeks instead of 12 or 15, but even that is a success. It beats the complete failure that occurs when you allow yourself to dip into the candy bowl or the cookie jar, begin to feel disgusted with yourself for having blown your diet, and then let all hell break loose. (*Safe fruits* are built in to the diet at levels of 1200 calories and above, without exceeding calorie limits.)

It is very important, however, that you choose only ONE safe fruit to be your ally during the Rotation Diet. Be sure, of course, to eat the different fruits that are included in the basic diet plan for each day's menu because they have been selected to provide you with adequate vitamins and minerals. However, if you add variety in your safe fruits, which you can eat at any time, you may stimulate your appetite. So, follow my advice: choose just one safe fruit from the following list. Use it as your snack food when it is called for at calorie levels of 1200 and above, and as an insurance or "fallback" food to be used whenever it is needed to prevent dangerous deviations from the Rotation Diet.

Be sure to think of your safe fruit as your ally. Pick one of the fruits in the short list below that you really do like. Have "friendly" feelings toward it! I think of fruit as one of Mother Nature's most enjoyable gifts to mankind—the word *fruit* comes from a Latin word meaning enjoyment or to enjoy. I know that I am going to stay slim and healthy every time I substitute a piece of fruit for one of man's enticing, but less healthful, junk-food creations! (If you are interested in determining more exact caloric values for each of these fruits, see Appendix A. I have restricted my list to fruits that are more generally available, but almost any fresh fruit will do.)

apple	orange
berries	peach
grapefruit	pineapple
melon	tangerine

ALLOWABLE BEVERAGES

You must have eight 8-ounce glasses of water each day. Water facilitates weight loss and helps you to stay healthy and regular when you are on a diet. Use ice water with a piece of lemon or lime if you find it difficult to drink the required amount, or use seltzer.

Avoid artificially sweetened beverages (see discussion on page 100). Up to two cups of coffee or tea are permitted, black coffee preferred. If you can't drink it black, a teaspoon of Half-and-Half will only add about 8 calories. You can also use herb teas in moderation, but I would avoid, for daily use, those that have laxative qualities. Try low-salt bouillons for a change (or make your own with meat or vegetable stock and added vegetables; see one of my recipes on page 69).

FOOD PREPARATION AND SIZE OF SERVINGS

Prepare your food simply without adding fat during the 600-calorie rotation, and use only the very small amounts of fat prescribed in the 900- and 1200-calorie rotations. Learn to use herbs and spices in place of salt (see discussion of salt below).

I have developed many recipes to illustrate delicious ways of preparing foods with few added fat calories. Recipes and serving suggestions are provided for all of the items on the Rotation Diet that are followed by an asterisk. (Recipes for the basic Rotation Diet begin on page 62.)

The correct serving sizes in either weight or volume are given both with the menus and with my recipes, and the calories in each serving are given with the recipes.

However, if you dislike weighing, measuring, and counting calories as much as I do, then, for convenience, all you need to remember when you prepare foods your own way, or when eating out, is that you will tend to be within the dietary guidelines when you choose standard, or moderate, "restaurant" portions such as you will find at a cafeteria.

If you do not have a good idea of serving sizes, it is worth your buying a scale and other measuring implements and measuring for a few days. Then you will have portion sizes stored in your memory, and you can discontinue the practice.

Standard Portions for Vegetables

Generally, a standard portion for vegetables (other than *free vegetables*) is a ½ cup. Some vegetables have so few calories that standard portions are as large as 1 cup. You will see which vegetables fall into this category as you follow the diet. And, of course, some vegetables are unlimited.

Standard Portions for Meat, Fish, and Fowl

For meat, fish, and fowl, a standard portion to fit the Rotation Diet plans for women during the 600/900 rotations is generally 3 ounces cooked weight (about 4 ounces raw). (Exceptions are noted in the daily menus.) Portions for women go up to either 4½ ounces or 6 ounces cooked (about 6 to 8 ounces raw) on the 1200-calorie rotation.

Portions for men are either 4½ or 6 ounces cooked weight (6 to 8 ounces raw) on their 1200-calorie rotations, and 6 ounces cooked (about 8 ounces raw) the 1500- and 1800-calorie rotations. (The variation in the recommended portions depends in part on what is on the rest of the day's menu, and the calories in the meat or fish itself.)

Standard Portions for Grain Foods

Among grains, 1 slice of bread = 1 ounce of dry cereal = ½ cup of rice = 5 whole-wheat crackers.

Standard Portions for Milk Products

Among milk products, 8 ounces of low-fat milk = 1 ounce of hard cheese = ½ cup of low-fat cottage cheese.

SNACKS

During the 600/900-calorie rotations for women, any snacks except for *free vegetables* will add enough calories to slow your weight loss slightly. However, should you feel uncomfortably hungry, I do urge you to use your *safe fruit* as a snack during this time. The slowdown in your rate of weight loss will be negligible compared to what will happen if you use anything other than your safe fruit. Remember, free vegetables and your safe fruit are your insurance policy. Use them and *guarantee* your weight loss.

Snacks (*safe fruits*) are included in all menus of 1200 calories and higher. It is not obligatory for you to eat all of these snacks, but when you reach the level of 1200 calories or higher, you should experiment with having one at mid-morning, at mid-afternoon, and at bedtime. As I indicated, I never went to bed hungry. And, after a grapefruit snack at bedtime, I always slept well, without waking up famished in the middle of the night.

Most persons who learn to eat healthful snacks during the Rotation Diet and then continue to do so during maintenance (eating fruits, vegetables, and low-calorie grains such as unbuttered popcorn in place of junk food) find it easier to control their weight in the long run. I normally nibble on fruit throughout the day. To be sure that you are not tempted to overeat and interfere with your rate of loss during the three weeks of the Rotation Diet, I suggest that you stick with your safe fruit as your only snack during this time. This will ensure that you stay well within the calorie guidelines. We will add more variety in the maintenance diet.

SUBSTITUTIONS

Women will do best to make as few substitutions as possible during the week they use the 600/900-calorie rotations. Even at this low intake, the diet has been designed to supply, insofar as possible, Recommended Dietary Allowances of the major vitamins and minerals, and to preserve your electrolyte balance (which affects heart rhythm). You can, of course, add free vegetables and your safe fruit. You can be somewhat more flexible during the 1200-calorie rotation, provided you make substitutions in accordance with certain dietary principles. Both men and women can have great flexibility at intakes of 1500 calories or higher. If you need to make substitutions in any of the menus, whether because of lack of availability of certain foods or because you don't like them, please read the section on making substitutions, which begins on page 114.

AN IMPORTANT WORD ABOUT SALT

The use of salt will impede your weight loss. Either use no salt at all in food preparation or, as I suggest in my recipes, add only the smallest amount, to taste. Many persons find they can cut back on salt considerably if they wait until after their food is cooked before adding any. Soy sauce is also somewhat high in sodium (about one-seventh the concentration of salt granules, or about 285 milligrams per teaspoon, compared with 2000 to 2200 milligrams for salt). Therefore, do not exceed the amounts called for when I suggest the use of soy sauce in my recipes. Also look for reduced-sodium soy sauces, which are widely available and taste just as good.

If you generally use salt, by all means try my recipe for Herb Salt (page 97). Herb Salt has one-seventh the amount of sodium in plain salt, which means that it has far less sodium in it than many commercially blended salt substitutes. Whereas just one-eighth teaspoon of salt has between 250 and 275 milligrams of sodium, Herb Salt has about 40 milligrams. Although Herb Salt has the same relative proportion of sodium to salt as does regular soy sauce, it is safer to use than soy sauce because you will tend to use much less of it. (Some salt substitutes completely replace the sodium component with potassium, but they tend not to taste nearly as good as Herb Salt.)

A cup of commercially prepared soup, such as mushroom, may contain nearly 1000 milligrams of sodium—in *one cup!* Ditto for a single serving of a frozen diet-dinner main course. As in the case of a pickle, that much sodium can lead to pounds of water retention.

Since my menus often call for crackers, look for the low-salt or no-salt varieties (see page 64 for suggestions).

Many packagers of foods (canned and frozen) have taken note of the new salt consciousness and now label some products "no salt added." You may wish to try some of these.

THE COUPLES ROTATION DIET

Although we designed separate menus for women and men, couples can use the Rotation Diet together. To do this, men use the basic Rotation Diet for women and add approximately 600 calories each day, throughout the twenty-one days.

Weeks 1 and 3

For best results, in Weeks 1 and 3 men use the Rotation Diet for women and add all of the following each day:

  2 more grain servings (bread, cereal, or crackers)
  50 percent larger portions of meat, fish, or fowl
  1 tablespoon of butter, oil, or regular salad dressing
  3 safe fruits

This is the healthiest way to add the 600-calorie difference required by men when they use the Rotation Diet for women during Weeks 1 and 3.

Week 2

In Week 2, when women are at approximately 1200 calories and men at 1800 calories, men have a tremendous amount of flexibility. Since the 1200-calorie diet for women has been designed to provide the RDAs of essential vitamins and minerals, a man could add 600 calories to the Rotation Diet for women in many different ways and still end up with a nutritious diet. For best results during Week 2, men should use the menu for women (which already includes three safe fruits and 1 tablespoon of fat for spread or seasoning) and add all of the following each day:

  2 more grain servings (bread, cereal, or crackers)
  50 percent larger portions of vegetables and main dishes

This will bring men up to about 1700 calories a day. The difference on the underside is due to the recipes in the male diet for Week 2 having slightly more fat in their preparation than the Week 2 recipes for women. This results from our intent to follow the nutritional guidelines of the United States Senate Committee on Nutrition and Human Needs in all daily menus of 1200 calories and over. In relation to total calories, these guidelines call for approximately 55 to 60 percent from carbohydrate, 25 to 30 percent from fat, and about 15 percent from protein. Thus, as calorie levels increase, men can have more of every nutrient. Including fat! But I wouldn't overdo it.

And women: please note that the Week 2 menus and the suggested recipes in the men's version of the Rotation Diet are very likely to be close to maintenance menus and recipes for you. I will be discussing the use of the men's menus in the transition to maintenance in Chapter 8.

ADVICE FOR SINGLES AND FOR THE DIETER WITH A FAMILY

For Singles

I know it is hard for single persons to go on a diet and cook for themselves alone, perhaps even harder than eating nutritiously as a single person when not on a reducing diet. Every time my wife goes on the road to perform and I am alone at home for days or weeks at a time, I find myself not wishing to cook well-rounded meals. But it can be done, and done easily, with just a little planning.

The best way, I think, is to cook up servings for two (cut recipes for four in half) and refrigerate or freeze the unused portions. You will be using the same foods again later in the diet, so you will already have them on hand. Most foods will keep well for three to five days in the refrigerator, and for months, of course, in the freezer. Cover appropriately for the refrigerator, and with freezer wrap for the freezer. You may also do the recipe for four and then freeze the food in separate, serving-size packages. That will save you time and bother in the future. We do a good deal of this large-batch cooking on weekends, and the remains serve us well during the coming week, when my wife and I both get home late from work and a bit too tired to cook a full meal from scratch.

For the Dieter with a Family

Whenever possible, use the basic menu in large enough amounts to feed everyone, adding any fattening seasonings later and separately for the family. Often this doesn't work, at first, because many members of the family are not accustomed to eating a nutritious diet! They will want different foods, turning up their noses at the vegetables, and insisting on fried dishes or other foods not on the diet, with lots of added fat or sugar. A microwave oven is a great gift on these occasions, since you can make your own vegetables in a couple of minutes. You may have to prepare your own menu separately—the plain-cooking style for the Rotation Diet will make it easier than if you try to follow elaborate methods of food preparation.

But if you plan in advance, I think you can reconcile the way you need to eat to lose weight quickly with the way your family likes the food prepared. Take a look at the menus, and see if you can make each evening's meal with your main dish held to the side while you add whatever your family wants to make it more enticing (if less nutritious) for them. And, if necessary, make your meals, or even some of your family's meals, in advance, on a weekend. Use serving sizes that will get you through the coming week or weeks, and freeze them.

Remember once again my advice to sit down for half an hour before you begin the Rotation Diet and figure out what it will take for you to approach perfection, given your particular life situation. If you talk it over with your family, explaining exactly what you will need to do for the next three weeks, I think you can get their help and cooperation. Lay the menus for the Rotation Diet before them, and discuss what it will take to keep everybody happy as you lose weight.

COPY (OR CUT OUT) YOUR PERSONAL
POCKET EDITION OF THE ROTATION DIET

For your convenience in following the Rotation Diet, I have designed a Pocket Edition of the menus that I am about to give you. The Pocket Edition for women will be found beginning on page 236, and the one for men on page 245. You can photocopy the Pocket Edition and carry it with you to help you select your foods throughout each day. You can show it to your friends when they begin to marvel at your weight loss (but, if your friends decide to go on the Rotation Diet with you, make sure they follow the instructions in the Pocket Edition). In case a photocopier is not easily available to you, the pages of the Pocket Edition are arranged so that you can cut them out of the book without damaging the other contents.

THE COMPLETE ROTATION DIET PLAN
MENUS FOR WOMEN

Additional information on serving sizes, *with caloric values,* will be found with the recipes that accompany all items followed by an asterisk. Do check out these excellent recipes. They illustrate that low-calorie cooking does not have to lead to boredom and deprivation.

Week 1

In the case of couples who wish to use the Rotation Diet together, men may use the basic diet plan for women with the addition of all of the following each day:

    2 more grain servings (bread, cereal, or crackers)
    50 percent larger portions of meat, fish, or fowl
    1 tablespoon of butter, oil, or regular salad dressing
    3 safe fruits

The calorie goal for men is 1200 calories for the first three days, and 1500 calories for the next four.

DAY 1

Breakfast: ½ grapefruit, 1 slice of whole-wheat bread and 1 slice of cheese (1 ounce, see Mexican Cheese Toast*), no-cal beverage
Lunch: 1 scoop of salmon (2 ounces canned in water, see Salmon with Herbs*), unlimited free vegetables, 5 whole-wheat crackers, no-cal beverage
Dinner: Baked Chicken* (3 ounces cooked), 1 serving each of cauliflower* (1 cup) and beets* (½ cup), 1 apple, no-cal beverage

DAY 2

Breakfast: ½ banana, 1 ounce of high-fiber cereal (see page 65), 8 ounces of skim or low-fat milk, no-cal beverage

Lunch: 1 scoop of low-fat cottage cheese (4 ounces, see Cottage Cheese Plus*), unlimited free vegetables, 1 slice of whole-wheat bread, no-cal beverage

Dinner: Poached Fish Fillet* (3 ounces, cooked), 1 serving each of broccoli* (1 cup) and carrots* (½ cup), ½ grapefruit, no-cal beverage

DAY 3

Breakfast: 1 slice of whole-wheat bread, 1 tablespoon of peanut butter, 1 apple, no-cal beverage

Lunch: Luncheon Tuna Vinaigrette* (2 ounces packed in water or 3 medium sardines from Sardines Vinaigrette*), 5 whole-wheat crackers, unlimited free vegetables, no-cal beverage

Dinner: Beefsteak or hamburger patty (3 ounces cooked, see Steak and Hamburger Teriyaki Style*), 1 cup of asparagus,* 1 cup of Dinner Salad,* No-Cal Salad Dressing,* 1 slice of cheese (1 ounce), 1 orange, no-cal beverage

DAY 4

Breakfast: ½ banana, 1 ounce of high-fiber cereal (see page 65), 8 ounces of skim or low-fat milk, no-cal beverage

Lunch: Tuna Salad* (with 2 ounces of water-packed tuna), unlimited free vegetables, 2 slices of whole-wheat bread, 1 teaspoon of mayonnaise or Lo-Cal Salad Dressing,* ½ grapefruit, no-cal beverage

Dinner: Baked Chicken* (3 ounces cooked), ½ cup of carrots,* 1 cup of Dinner Salad,* 1 slice of cheese (1 ounce), 1 apple, no-cal beverage

DAY 5

Breakfast: 1 cup of berries, 1 serving of low-fat cottage cheese (4 ounces, see Cottage Cheese Plus*), 5 whole-wheat crackers, no-cal beverage

Lunch: Sardines Vinaigrette* (3 medium; or Tuna Vinaigrette,* 2 ounces canned in water), unlimited free vegetables, 2 slices of whole-wheat bread, 1 teaspoon of mayonnaise or Lo-Cal Salad Dressing,* ½ grapefruit, no-cal beverage

Dinner: Beefsteak or hamburger patty (3 ounces cooked, see Steak and Hamburger Teriyaki Style*), 1 serving each of green beans* (½ cup) and broccoli* (1 cup), 1 slice of cheese (1 ounce), 1 apple, no-cal beverage

DAY 6

Breakfast: ½ cantaloupe, 1 slice of cheese (1 ounce) and 1 slice of whole-wheat bread (see Mexican Cheese Toast*), no-cal beverage

Lunch: 1 hard-boiled egg (see Curried Unstuffed Hard-boiled Egg*), unlimited free vegetables, 2 slices of whole-wheat bread, 1 teaspoon of mayonnaise or Lo-Cal Salad Dressing,* ½ grapefruit, no-cal beverage

Dinner: Poached (or Baked) Fish Fillet* (3 ounces), 1 serving each of asparagus* (1 cup) and green peas* (½ cup), 1 apple, no-cal beverage

DAY 7

Breakfast: ½ banana, 1 ounce of high-fiber cereal (see page 65), 8 ounces of skim or low-fat milk, no-cal beverage

Lunch: 1 cup of berries, 1 serving of low-fat cottage cheese (4 ounces, see Cottage Cheese Plus*), 2 slices of whole-wheat bread, no-cal beverage

Dinner: Baked Chicken* (3 ounces cooked), 1 serving each of cauliflower* (1 cup) and carrots* (½ cup), 1 apple, no-cal beverage

Week 2

In Week 2 women may add a mid-morning, a mid-afternoon, and an evening snack, intentionally incorporating three servings of your *safe fruit.* It is not obligatory to include all of these snacks in addition to the menus below, but they are permitted within the 1200-calorie limits for this week. You may also add 1 tablespoon of butter, margarine, oil, or regular salad dressing to your diet each day. Use it for cooking or as a spread.

For couples' use, men should add all of the following each day to the daily menus of the Rotation Diet for women, below.

2 more grain servings (bread, cereal, or crackers)
50 percent larger portions of vegetables and main courses

Optional for men: another tablespoon of fat for spread or seasoning. The calorie goal for males is 1800 per day throughout Week 2. Additional information on serving sizes, *with caloric values,* will be found with the recipes.

DAY 8

Breakfast: ½ grapefruit, 1 slice of whole-wheat bread, 1 tablespoon of peanut butter, 8 ounces of skim or low-fat milk, no-cal beverage

Lunch: large fruit salad (about 2 cups, see Creative Fruit Salad*), 1 slice of cheese (1 ounce), 5 whole-wheat crackers, no-cal beverage

Dinner: salmon steak (4½ ounces, see Royal Indian Salmon*), 1 serving of Peas and Baby Onions* (½ cup), 1 cup of Dinner Salad,* no-cal beverage

DAY 9

Breakfast: ½ banana, 1 ounce of high-fiber cereal (see page 65), 8 ounces of skim or low-fat milk, no-cal beverage

Lunch: large chef salad (1 ounce each of cheese and turkey plus any salad vegetables, see Creative Chef Salad*), 5 whole-wheat crackers, Lo-Cal Salad Dressing,* no-cal beverage

Dinner: chicken (4½ ounces cooked, see Chicken Tomasi* for something special tonight), 1 small baked potato (3½ ounces), green beans (1 cup, or try Green Beans Almondine*), 1 slice of cheese (1 ounce), 1 apple, no-cal beverage

DAY 10

Breakfast: sliced fresh fruit of your choice (1 cup), 1 serving of low-fat cottage cheese (4 ounces), 1 slice of whole-wheat bread, no-cal beverage

Lunch: sandwich (2 ounces of meat or cheese, or see Combination Sandwich*), unlimited free vegetables, 1 orange, no-cal beverage

Dinner: Stir-Fry Vegetables* (2 cups), Brown or Wild Rice* (½ cup), 2 tablespoons of grated cheese, 1 apple, no-cal beverage

DAY 11

Breakfast: 1 cup of fresh pineapple (or other fresh fruit), 1 slice of cheese (1 ounce), 1 slice of whole-wheat bread, no-cal beverage

Lunch: Spinach Salad* (large 2–3 cups, with sliced mushrooms, green peppers, and chopped egg), Lo-Cal Salad Dressing,* 1 apple or pear, 1 slice of cheese (1 ounce), no-cal beverage

Dinner: steak (6 ounces, see Steak Flamed in Brandy* or Marinated Flank Steak*), 1 small baked potato (3½ ounces), Braised Carrots and Celery* (1 cup), ½ grapefruit, no-cal beverage

DAY 12

Breakfast: sliced fruit (½ cup), 1 ounce of high-fiber cereal (see page 65), 8 ounces of skim or low-fat milk, no-cal beverage

Lunch: Tuna Salad* or Sardines Vinaigrette* (with 3 ounces of water-packed tuna or 4–5 medium sardines), unlimited free vegetables plus sliced tomato and green pepper, Lo-Cal Salad Dressing,* 1 slice of whole-wheat bread, no-cal beverage

Dinner: Herbed Pork* (6 ounces), ½ baked Acorn Squash,* Broccoli with Black Olives* (1 cup of broccoli), ½ grapefruit, no-cal beverage

DAY **13**

Breakfast:	½ melon, 1 hard- or soft-boiled egg, 1 slice of whole-wheat bread, no-cal beverage
Lunch:	dieter's special: ground-beef patty (4½ ounces cooked), 1 serving of low-fat cottage cheese (4 ounces), sliced tomato and unlimited free vegetables, Lo-Cal Salad Dressing,* no-cal beverage
Dinner:	My Favorite Pasta* (1 cup, plus choice of sauce), 2 tablespoons of Parmesan cheese, 1 cup of Dinner Salad,* choice of 1 fresh fruit, no-cal beverage

DAY **14**

Breakfast:	½ grapefruit, 1 cup of oatmeal, 2 tablespoons of raisins, dash of cinnamon, 4 ounces of skim or low-fat milk, no-cal beverage
Lunch:	toasted open-faced sandwich (try Mexican Bean Spread,* 1 slice of cheese, and sliced tomato, or see Day 10 for a regular sandwich), unlimited free vegetables, 1 cup of assorted sliced fresh fruit, no-cal beverage
Dinner:	Pot Roast of Beef, Italian Style* (4 ounces of meat, cooked, including vegetables), 1 cup of Dinner Salad,* Lo-Cal Salad Dressing,* 1 slice of cheese (1 ounce), 1 apple, no-cal beverage

Week 3

Repeat the menus of Week 1, or use the Alternate Menus in Chapter 12 for the 600- and 900-calorie rotations.

When you finish your twenty-one days on the Rotation Diet, BE VERY SURE THAT YOU FOLLOW MY DIRECTIONS FOR MAKING A TRANSITION TO MAINTENANCE IN WEEK 4 (CHAPTER 8).

THE COMPLETE ROTATION DIET PLAN
MENUS FOR MEN

Week 1

Men may incorporate three *safe fruit* snacks each day within calorie guidelines throughout the Rotation Diet, but it is not obligatory. You may also add 1 tablespoon of butter, margarine, or regular salad dressing (in place of lo-cal) to each day's menu and remain within the calorie limits.

DAY 1

Breakfast: ½ banana, 1 ounce of high-fiber cereal (see page 65), 8 ounces of skim or low-fat milk, no-cal beverage

Lunch: large chef salad (1 ounce each of cheese and turkey, plus any salad vegetables, see Creative Chef Salad*), Lo-Cal Salad Dressing,* 5 whole-wheat crackers, no-cal beverage

Dinner: Baked Chicken* (4½ ounces cooked), 1 small baked potato (3½ ounces), 1 serving of green beans* (1 cup), 1 apple, 1 slice of cheese (1 ounce), no-cal beverage

DAY 2

Breakfast: ½ grapefruit, 1 slice of whole-wheat bread, 1 tablespoon of peanut butter, 8 ounces of skim or low-fat milk, no-cal beverage

Lunch: large fruit salad (about 2 cups, see Creative Fruit Salad*), 1 slice of cheese (1 ounce), 5 whole-wheat crackers, no-cal beverage

Dinner: Poached (or Baked) Fish Fillet* (6 ounces cooked), 1 serving of Green Peas and Baby Onions* (½ cup), Dinner Salad* (1 cup), Lo-Cal Salad Dressing,* no-cal beverage

DAY **3**

Breakfast: 1 cup of sliced fruit (your choice), 1 serving of low-fat cottage cheese (4 ounces), 1 slice of whole-wheat bread, no-cal beverage

Lunch: Combination Sandwich* (2 ounces of meat or cheese), unlimited free vegetables, 1 orange, no-cal beverage

Dinner: Stir-Fry Vegetables* (2 cups), Brown or Wild Rice* (½ cup), 2 tablespoons of grated cheese, 1 apple, no-cal beverage

DAY **4**

Breakfast: 1 cup of berries, 1½ ounces of high-fiber cereal (see page 65), 8 ounces of skim or low-fat milk, 1 slice of whole-wheat bread, 1 teaspoon of preserves, no-cal beverage

Lunch: Spinach Salad* (large 2–3 cups, with sliced mushrooms, green peppers, chopped egg, and Lo-Cal Salad Dressing*), 5 whole-wheat crackers, 1 apple or pear, no-cal beverage

Dinner: ½ grapefruit, steak (6 ounces cooked, see Steak Flamed in Brandy* or Marinated Flank Steak*), 1 small baked potato (3½ ounces), Braised Carrots and Celery* (1 cup), no-cal beverage

DAY **5**

Breakfast: ½ melon, 1 hard- or soft-boiled egg, 2 slices of whole-wheat bread, 1 teaspoon of preserves, no-cal beverage

Lunch: ground-beef patty (4½ ounces cooked, see Steak and Hamburger Teriyaki Style*), 1 serving of low-fat cottage cheese (4 ounces), unlimited free vegetables, 1 slice of whole-wheat bread, 1 serving of fruit (your choice), no-cal beverage

Dinner: My Favorite Pasta* (1 cup, plus choice of sauce), 4 tablespoons of grated Parmesan cheese, Dinner Salad* (1 cup), Lo-Cal Salad Dressing,* ½ grapefruit, no-cal beverage

DAY 6

Breakfast: 1 cup of sliced fruit, 1½ ounces of high-fiber cereal (see page 65), 1 slice of whole-wheat bread, 8 ounces of skim or low-fat milk, no-cal beverage

Lunch: Tuna Salad* or Sardines Vinaigrette* (3 ounces of water-packed tuna, or 4–5 medium sardines), unlimited free vegetables plus sliced tomato and green pepper, Lo-Cal Salad Dressing,* 2 slices of whole-wheat bread, no-cal beverage

Dinner: Herbed Pork* (6 ounces cooked), ½ baked Acorn Squash,* Broccoli with Black Olives* (1 cup of broccoli), 1 slice of whole-wheat bread, ½ grapefruit, no-cal beverage

DAY 7

Breakfast: ½ grapefruit, 1 cup of oatmeal, 2 tablespoons of raisins, dash of cinnamon, 4 ounces of skim or low-fat milk, no-cal beverage

Lunch: open-faced sandwich (2 portions, see Mexican Bean Spread,* with 1 slice of cheese and sliced tomato, or see Day 3 for a regular sandwich), unlimited free vegetables, Lo-Cal Salad Dressing,* 1 cup of assorted fresh fruit, no-cal beverage

Dinner: Pot Roast of Beef* (4 ounces of meat, including vegetables), Dinner Salad* (1 cup), Lo-Cal Salad Dressing,* 1 apple, no-cal beverage

Week 2

During Week 2 you can add 1 tablespoon of butter, margarine, or regular salad dressing to each day's menu, as well as the three *safe fruits*, and remain within the calorie limits.

DAY 8

Breakfast: ½ melon, 2 slices of whole-wheat bread, 2 slices of cheese (2 ounces), no-cal beverage

Lunch: Tuna-Salad Sandwich* (3 ounces of water-packed

tuna), unlimited free vegetables, 1 serving of fruit (your choice), no-cal beverage

Dinner: Baked Chicken* (6 ounces cooked), Spinach and Broccoli Casserole* (½ cup, or 1 cup of broccoli plainly prepared), ½ baked Acorn Squash,* 1 apple, 1 slice of cheese (1 ounce, if casserole recipe is not used), no-cal beverage

DAY 9

Breakfast: 1 cup of oatmeal, 2 tablespoons of raisins, dash of cinnamon, 4 ounces of skim or low-fat milk, 1 slice of whole-wheat bread, 1 teaspoon of preserves, no-cal beverage

Lunch: large fruit salad (2 cups, see Creative Fruit Salad*), 1 serving of low-fat cottage cheese (4 ounces), 5 whole-wheat crackers, no-cal beverage

Dinner: Baked (or Poached) Fish Fillet* (6 ounces), Baked Tomato* (½ tomato), 1 small baked potato (3½ ounces), Dinner Salad* (1 cup), 1 slice of cheese (1 ounce), 1 apple, no-cal beverage

DAY 10

Breakfast: 1 orange, 2 slices of whole-wheat bread, 2 slices of cheese (2 ounces), no-cal beverage

Lunch: Tuna Salad* (3 ounces of water-packed tuna) on greens with sliced tomatoes and green pepper, plus unlimited free vegetables, Lo-Cal Salad Dressing,* no-cal beverage

Dinner: Steak (6 ounces cooked, see Marinated Flank Steak* or Steak Flamed in Brandy*), Stir-Fry Spinach* (1 cup), 1 small baked potato (3½ ounces) with Cottage-Cheese Dressing* (or 2 tablespoons of sour cream), choice of 1 fruit, no-cal beverage

DAY 11

Breakfast: ½ melon, 1 serving of low-fat cottage cheese (4 ounces), 1 slice of whole-wheat bread, 1 teaspoon of preserves, no-cal beverage

Lunch: sandwich (2 ounces of meat or cheese; see Combination Sandwich*), unlimited free vegetables, Lo-Cal Salad Dressing,* no-cal beverage

Dinner: Baked Salmon* (6 ounces cooked, see Royal Indian Salmon*), Peas and Baby Onions* (½ cup), Dinner Salad* (1 cup), Lo-Cal Salad Dressing,* choice of 1 fruit, 1 slice of cheese (1 ounce), no-cal beverage

DAY 12

Breakfast: ½ grapefruit, 2 slices of whole-wheat bread, 1 tablespoon of peanut butter, 1 teaspoon of preserves, no-cal beverage

Lunch: 1 cup of soup (commercial or see Soups*), 10 whole-wheat crackers, 2 slices of cheese (2 ounces), unlimited free vegetables, Lo-Cal Salad Dressing,* no-cal beverage

Dinner: Veal Loaf* (or 6 ounces cooked, of lean meat of your choice), carrots* (½ cup), Dinner Salad* (1 cup), Lo-Cal Salad Dressing,* 1 apple, no-cal beverage

DAY 13

Breakfast: 1 cup of berries, 1½ ounces of high-fiber cereal (see page 65), 1 slice of whole-wheat bread, 1 teaspoon of preserves, 8 ounces of skim or low-fat milk, no-cal beverage

Lunch: large chef salad (1 ounce each of cheese and turkey, plus any salad vegetables, see Creative Chef Salad*), Lo-Cal Salad Dressing,* 5 whole-wheat crackers, no-cal beverage

Dinner: Baked Chicken* (6 ounces cooked, or try Almond Chicken*), 1 serving of Brown or Wild Rice* (½ cup), broccoli* (1 cup), 1 slice of cheese (1 ounce), 1 apple, no-cal beverage

DAY 14

Breakfast: choice of sliced fruit (1 cup), 1 serving of low-fat cottage cheese (4 ounces), 1 slice of whole-wheat bread, 1 teaspoon of preserves, no-cal beverage

Lunch: sandwich (2 ounces of meat or cheese, see Combination Sandwich*), unlimited free vegetables, Lo-Cal Salad Dressing,* ½ grapefruit, no-cal beverage

Dinner: fish of your choice (6 ounces cooked, or try Baked or Broiled Rainbow Trout*), Baked Tomato* (½ tomato), Green Beans with Chives* (1 cup, or use mushroom variation), 1 slice of whole-wheat bread, 1 slice of cheese (1 ounce), 1 fruit of your choice, no-cal beverage

Week 3

Repeat the menus of Week 1, or use the Alternate Menus in Chapter 12 for the 1200- and 1500-calorie rotations.

When you finish your twenty-one days on the Rotation Diet, BE VERY SURE THAT YOU FOLLOW MY DIRECTIONS FOR MAKING A TRANSITION TO MAINTENANCE IN WEEK 4 (CHAPTER 8).

RECIPES

The recipes and serving suggestions for the Rotation Diet are meant to illustrate that low-calorie cooking need not be boring and without taste. However, for simplicity's sake, you may prepare everything plain, or according to your own favorite recipes, provided you do not add fat, sugar, or anything else that will increase the calorie content appreciably.

To facilitate weight loss, do not use salt. However, if you must have a small amount of salt for flavoring, it is best to add it after cooking, at the table.

See my recipe for Herb Salt (page 97), which cuts out over 85 percent of the sodium. It's a great blend.

Except for *free vegetables,* be sure to adhere to the serving sizes recommended. And, of course, remember that you have a *safe fruit* that you can use to make sure you do not feel hungry.

Grains, Breads, Crackers, Cereals

I advise you to use either 100 percent whole-grain breads and crackers or breads and crackers that have as their primary ingredient a whole grain. If the primary ingredient is a whole grain, it will be listed first on the label of a commercial product.

Breads and crackers in the grocery store that say "100 percent whole wheat" and those listing only "whole-wheat flour" as the grain ingredient will be made entirely of whole grains. Blends will list other grains or types of flour.

I like breads made from whole-grain products because they offer a wider array of vitamins and minerals than the refined-grain products and three or more times the dietary fiber.

Most commercial whole-wheat breads contain about 65–70 calories per slice, and the usual whole-wheat cracker has about 17 calories (five whole-wheat crackers will be about 85 calories).

BREADS

Here are two outstanding whole-wheat breads that were developed especially for the Rotation Diet by one of Nashville's outstanding bakers and teachers of baking, Ms. Joyce Weingartner. As you will see when you try these recipes, blending a small amount of other flours with the primary whole-wheat flour provides a lighter, more attractive texture than can be obtained by using only whole-wheat flour. In addition, the use of other flours in small amounts increases the overall nutritional value of the bread, since the other flours have a different array of nutrients. Both of these breads are batter breads, which makes for quick and easy baking.

WHOLE-WHEAT BATTER BREAD

In a large mixing bowl combine:

    5 cups of whole-wheat flour
    ½ cup of barley flour (white can be substituted)
    ½ cup of soy flour

½ cup of sugar (you may mix ¼ cup of white and ¼ cup of brown)

1 tablespoon of salt (or just 2 teaspoons of salt, which we like, since it yields a slightly sweeter-tasting bread)

2 packages of dry yeast

Pour in 3½ cups of warm water and stir 200 strong strokes until blended

Mixing the ingredients should take at least 3 minutes until the flours are completely incorporated. This will yield a soft batter that is not to be kneaded.

With a wooden spoon, fill two 5-by-9-inch bread pans, which have been well greased. Push dough into the corners and smooth the top surface. A wet spoon helps this process.

Cover with a warm, wet towel and place in a draft-free area until the batter has doubled.

Preheat oven to 400 degrees and bake for 15 minutes.

Reduce heat to 350 degrees and continue baking for another 45 minutes.

To prevent the top of the bread from becoming too dark, you may cover it with foil for the last half-hour of baking.

Test each loaf for a hollow sound when you remove it from the oven and the pan. If the bread is soft on the bottom, return to the oven for about 10 additional minutes.

Remove bread from pans and place on a metal rack to cool, with a cloth over the bread.

Cool before serving.

Store in a plastic bag in the refrigerator if you will use it immediately (in a week, for example), or in a plastic bag in the freezer for longer periods.

Note: If you wish to have a bread that is 100 percent whole wheat, delete the barley and soy flours and use 6 cups of whole-wheat flour in this recipe.

OATMEAL BATTER BREAD

While proofing 2 packages of yeast in ¼ cup water to which have been added ¼ teaspoon of sugar and ¼ teaspoon of ginger:

Mix 2 cups of warm water with 1 cup of Quaker Oats (regular

kind), 1 tablespoon of butter, 1½ teaspoons of salt, and ⅓ cup of molasses.

Add the yeast mixture to the oats.

Stir in 2 cups of whole-wheat flour and stir 100 strong strokes to blend.

Add:

½ cup of soy flour
½ cup of white flour
¼ cup of wheat germ

Stir well after each addition.

Add an additional 1¼ cups of whole-wheat flour.

Stir well for 3 minutes so that all ingredients are completely blended. This will yield a soft, sticky batter, which is not to be kneaded.

Cover with a warm, wet cloth and place in a draft-free warm place until the batter has doubled—about 1 to 1¼ hours.

Stir down and spoon into three 7¼-by-3½-inch greased bread pans for small loaves, or into two 9-by-5-inch bread pans for larger loaves.

Cover with a wet cloth and allow to double in bulk (around 45 minutes).

When spooning the batter in, it helps to use a wet spoon to fill the pans and push the batter into the corners. The top will look like a plowed field, but this is not important to the taste.

Preheat oven to 350 degrees and bake for 55 minutes.

For a crusty bottom you may place the loaf on the rack of the oven for 5 minutes without the pan (optional).

Cool on a wire rack with a cloth over the bread before serving.

Store in a plastic bag in the refrigerator or for longer periods in the freezer.

CRACKERS

Many crackers contain a great deal of sodium, which will seriously slow your weight loss. Avoid saltines and soda crackers.

Check labels, and, if your store does not carry attractive crackers that have a whole grain listed as their first or only ingredient, choose those that list a whole grain, or bran, as a second ingredient. Venus-brand crackers (any variety) are good choices from this second category. Venus makes excellent no-salt-added crackers as well.

CEREALS

Here is a list of the relatively high-fiber cereals that I refer to in my menus:

40% Bran Flakes	Bran Buds	Wheat Chex
Shredded Wheat	Puffed Wheat	Bran Chex
Shredded Wheat 'N Bran	Oat Bran	Corn Bran
All Bran	Grape-Nuts	Oatmeal

If you have not been in the habit of eating a cereal that's relatively high in fiber, you might sample a variety in the new *Kellogg's Fiber Pack Assortment* and find one that you like. If you prefer a cereal that is relatively low in fiber, you can enhance the fiber content of your own favorite cereal with the addition of fresh fruit or with 2-3 tablespoons of All Bran or Bran Buds. For example, the *Special K Breakfast,* which was especially designed with weight management in mind, would be a good choice with fruit.

Milk and Milk Products

Skim milk has virtually no fat and contains about 80 calories per 8 ounces. Low-fat milk will contain about 100 calories for 1 percent butterfat content, and around 120 calories if it has a 2 percent butterfat content. I use low-fat milk because its fat content satisfies hunger for a much longer period of time than does skim milk (and I prefer the flavor).

CHEESE

Many herbs, seeds, and spices can be used to advantage with cheese. My favorite herbs are dillweed, rosemary, sage, and thyme. Seeds include caraway, celery, and dill. Certain spices can be sprinkled over cheddar, Monterey Jack, Swiss, or Halvarti cheese and then toasted on a slice of whole-wheat bread, in either a regular or microwave oven. This makes a tasty, toasted, open-faced sandwich for breakfast or lunch. The best spices for cheese toast include chili powder, cumin, or curry powder, plus a dash of cayenne pepper.

Be sure to control your serving size of cheese. Many varieties are high in sodium. Cheddar has about 200 milligrams per ounce, while blue has almost 400 milligrams per ounce. Monterey Jack, Muenster, Tilsit, and Swiss are among the lowest, at around 100 milligrams per ounce.

Try the following Mexican Cheese Toast when the diet calls for 1 slice (about 1 ounce) of cheese and 1 slice of whole-wheat bread.

MEXICAN CHEESE TOAST

1 ounce of cheese (cheddar, Monterey Jack, Swiss)
Chili powder
1 slice of whole-wheat bread
Dash of cayenne (optional)

Slice the cheese thinly so that it covers the bread. Sprinkle generously with chili powder and add a dash of cayenne if you like it hot. This takes less than a minute to melt in a microwave, or you can do it under a broiler, in which case it will take a little longer and bear watching.

Any time the menu calls for a slice of cheese and a slice of bread, you can combine them to make some form of cheese toast. Vary the recipe by using the other herbs and spices.

The average slice of bread is about 70 calories, while a slice of cheese (about 1 ounce in weight) will generally contain 100 calories. Thus, cheese toast will have approximately 170 calories.

COTTAGE CHEESE PLUS

Of course the Rotation Diet recommends cottage cheese as one of the dairy staples in its menus. Cottage cheese is a very good source of protein, carbohydrate, and calcium. I like cottage cheese with just about any fruit except citrus. If you don't care much for cottage cheese in its plain form, or soon get bored with it, try flavoring it with one or more of the herbs and spices I mentioned above to make Cottage Cheese Plus. Also, in addition to or instead of celery seed, I especially like to sprinkle my cottage cheese with either onion or garlic powder. If you can't get excited about cottage cheese, try Breakstone's Low-Fat Cottage Cheese. Participants in the Vanderbilt Weight Management Program rate Breakstone's a winner in all comparison tests.

Serving size is ½ cup, at about 90 calories per serving.

Eggs

CURRIED UNSTUFFED HARD-BOILED EGG

You can more than double the calories in deviled or stuffed eggs when you add those gobs of mayonnaise. It's unnecessary. Just sprinkle slices of hard-boiled egg with one or more of the following: curry or chili powder, cumin, onion powder, celery seeds, freshly ground black pepper. I find that any of these seasonings will satisfy my palate without adding mayonnaise or salt.

Serving size is 1 egg, at about 80 calories per egg.

Sandwiches

COMBINATION SANDWICH

The label "Combination Sandwich" refers to any combination of ingredients between 2 slices of bread, such as ham (or any slice of meat) and cheese, or spreads with vegetables or cheese.

The way to prepare sandwiches with limited calories is to use lean cuts of meat or fowl, and only limited amounts of dressing. Two slices of bread, with 1 ounce each of meat and cheese, will contain about 295 calories. Mayonnaise is about 33 calories a teaspoon, catsup is 16 calories a tablespoon, and mustard is negligible. Add *free vegetables* and you have a satisfying lunch for about 350 calories. (Compare the calorie content of this lunch with the 650 or so calories you obtain in the typical fast-food hamburger sandwich. The fast-food hamburger can have as much as five times the fat content of your lean slice of meat, and three to six times more mayonnaise or salad dressing will be used to enhance the flavor.)

For variety, try one of the following spreads. They make especially attractive open-faced sandwiches. Serve with sprouts, or a slice of tomato or cheese, and broil in the oven for a hot sandwich.

Meat Spread

½ pound of cooked meat or fowl	2 tablespoons of soy flour
1 small onion, diced	Herb Salt (p. 97)
¼ cup of wheat germ (or cooked red beans)	Freshly ground black pepper

Blend all ingredients in a food processor. Moisten as needed with catsup or salad dressing.

Makes about 1¼ cups; serving size is about 2 ounces, or ¼ cup, at about 95 calories per serving.

Crab-Meat Spread

1 cup of crab meat	½ green pepper, diced
½ cup of celery, diced	1 cup of sprouts
1 small onion, diced	1 cup of low-fat cottage cheese
Herb Salt to taste (p. 97)	

Blend with enough salad dressing to moisten. Makes about 3 cups; serving size is about 2 ounces, or ¼ cup, at about 35 calories per serving.

Mexican Bean Spread

This is one of my favorites. It can substitute for a Mexican bean dip, and it is great broiled in the oven covered with a slice of cheese, or tomato, and sprinkled with oregano.

1 can of dark-red kidney beans	Herb Salt (p. 97)
1 small onion	Freshly ground black pepper
3 tablespoons of catsup	
⅛ teaspoon of cayenne pepper	

Blend in a food processor, adding more catsup if needed for desired consistency.

Makes about 1½ cups; serving size is about 2 ounces, or ¼ cup, at about 90 calories per serving.

TUNA- OR SALMON-SALAD SANDWICH

See the recipe for tuna or salmon salad on page 72. With 2 slices of bread, lettuce, and/or sprouts, plus ¼ of the salad recipe, a typical sandwich will contain between 260 and 325 calories, depending upon the amount of mayonnaise used.

Soups

SOUP BASE

This is the basic stock that I use for making soup of various kinds, rice, and boiled potatoes. It is excellent for soaking and cooking beans. By adding only a minimal amount of salt, you can keep the sodium content of your own stock at a fraction of what is contained in commercial soups and bouillons.

Save all chicken and turkey giblets (necks, hearts, gizzards, but *not* livers) and freeze immediately, first trimming skin and any fat from the necks. Hold in your freezer until you have accumulated the parts of 4 to 6 birds. Then:

Place giblets in a deep soup kettle, with enough water to cover (about 8 to 10 cups). Bring to a boil and skim as necessary. When finally clear of scum, add:

1 large bay leaf
1 teaspoon each of rosemary, sage, thyme, and tarragon
2 large stalks of celery, in 2-inch pieces (include leaves)

Salt and pepper to taste
1 large onion, coarsely chopped
2 large carrots, in 2-inch pieces

Throw in any other greens or wilted vegetables you have hanging out in your refrigerator (except for cabbage, broccoli, or cauliflower).

Bring to boil once again, then reduce heat and simmer for at least 2 hours.

Separate giblets and vegetables from water. Blend vegetables and return to stock. Save giblets for low-calorie snacks.

Freeze the stock in 2- to 4-cup plastic containers and use as needed.

THURSDAY'S VEGETABLE SOUP

This soup bears the name it does because I made it for the first time on a Thursday, a day before I was about to do a television show on low-calorie cooking, when the temperature was near zero outdoors. What could be better than a hot cup of soup on such a day?

To 1 cup of soup stock (or commercial low-salt bouillon), throw in a quartered onion, sliced carrot, and a sliced stalk of celery, plus anything else in the way of vegetables that you have left over in the refrigerator (red cabbage will give it a delightful red tint).

Add seasonings to taste—for example, thyme, a few sprigs of rosemary, a touch of parsley, etc.

Each serving of 1 cup contains about 15 to 20 calories; depending on how many vegetables you throw in, you can end up with 2 or 3 cups, at about 40 or 60 calories for the total.

This soup is another food that you can use almost as freely as a *free vegetable* (some of the vegetables that you use may be more than 10 calories a serving).

You can make the soup a little heartier by using some potatoes, and I strongly suggest that you do occasionally. This will make the soup even more filling and satisfy your hunger for longer periods. A small (3½-ounce) potato will add only 90 calories to the entire recipe.

Salads

CREATIVE FRUIT SALAD

This is called Creative Fruit Salad because you use whatever fruits you have on hand, cut them up into chunks, sprinkle with lemon juice to keep the fruit looking fresh and to add a bit of tang, and then add 1 tablespoon of ONE of any of the following:

> grated coconut
> chopped unsalted nuts (of any kind)
> raisins or chopped dates

Add a sprinkle of any of the following spices:

> cinnamon   ginger
> nutmeg   anise
> allspice   cardamom

A main-course serving is 2 cups of any combination of fresh fruits plus 1 tablespoon of nuts or raisins. Average calories: about 200 per serving.

CREATIVE CHEF SALAD

Several large leaves of romaine
¼ head of any lettuce, shredded
¼ cup of red cabbage, shredded
¼ cup of shaved carrots
1 ounce of Swiss cheese, cut in narrow strips
1 ounce of white-meat turkey or chicken, in strips

Plus choice of additional vegetables
1 egg, quartered (optional)
1 tomato, quartered
1 slice of green pepper
Lo-Cal Salad Dressing (p. 75)
Herb Salt (p. 97)
Freshly ground black pepper

Arrange your selections attractively on the romaine and use 1 to 2 tablespoons of dressing.

The calorie content of this salad will range from 300 to 400, depending on whether you include the egg, and the amount of dressing you use.

DINNER SALAD

For each portion, use:

½ carrot, thinly sliced
1 stalk of celery, thinly sliced or
¼ green pepper, diced
lettuce or greens (*free vegetables*)

¼ cup of shredded red cabbage or
4 sliced mushrooms
2 thin slices of sweet red onion

A dinner sized salad bowl of this mixture will contain about 40 calories. Use with No- or Lo-Cal Salad Dressing (p. 75) and flavor with Herb Salt (p. 97) if you like.

TUNA OR SALMON SALAD

1 6½-ounce can of water-packed tuna or salmon

1 large carrot
2 stalks of celery

Blend in a food processor or blender, adding enough salad dressing or mayonnaise for desired consistency. If you prefer to do the blending by hand, the carrot and celery should be sliced thin, or chopped. Serve with lettuce and tomato, or with 2 slices of bread and sprouts as a sandwich.

Blended with 1 tablespoon of mayonnaise, this makes 3 tuna-salad portions at 136 calories each. If you leave out the mayonnaise, the calories per serving are 103. For salmon-salad portions of the same size, add 30 calories.

SALMON WITH HERBS

Even canned salmon can be interesting when it's dressed in its most complementary herbs. My favorites are thyme, marjoram, or sage—just a dash or two of each. Celery seed goes well, too, and so does the mustard vinaigrette dressing I suggest below for the sardines (a bit of mustard and a drop of lemon juice or vinegar). Serve with toast, whole-wheat crackers, and/or a leaf of romaine.

Serving size is 3 ounces, at 156 calories per serving.

SARDINES VINAIGRETTE

I include sardines because they are an excellent low-calorie source of protein and calcium, even when packed in oil. Their nutritional value makes them an excellent addition to the 600/900-calorie rotations. Just drain, and top with a bit of Dijon mustard and a drop of lemon juice or vinegar. Serve on a leaf or two of romaine, and garnish with any of your *free vegetables*.

Serving size is 2 ounces, or about 3 medium-sized sardines, at 88 calories per serving.

SPINACH SALAD

For each serving:

2 cups of fresh spinach, trimmed
3 large mushrooms, sliced
½ hard-boiled egg, chopped
1 Bermuda onion, sliced (optional)

3 slices of green pepper
Lo-cal dressing of your choice (or see p. 75)

Arrange spinach on a large platter, and then layer the other vegetables over it in an attractive manner—a spinach salad is one of the most pleasant salads to behold, especially if you do choose to add a few slices of Bermuda onion.

Contains about 115 calories per serving, including the egg. Add 33 calories per tablespoon of Lo-Cal Salad Dressing (p. 75), or check the bottle of any lo-cal dressing of your own. If you wish to keep the calories down, use No-Cal Salad Dressing (p. 75).

LUNCHEON TUNA VINAIGRETTE

I prefer my tuna plain with a few drops of fresh lemon juice or wine vinegar. For extra zest, try canned, water-packed tuna with tarragon vinegar (you can buy this commercially) or use my recipe for No-Cal Salad Dressing below, with the addition of tarragon.

Serving size is 3 ounces at 120 calories per serving.

Salad Dressings

COTTAGE-CHEESE DRESSING

½ cup of low-fat cottage cheese
½ cup of plain low-fat yogurt
½ green pepper, chopped
4 radishes, sliced
2 tablespoons of chives
1 tablespoon of poppy seeds
Herb Salt to taste

Mix in a blender or food processor. It is excellent with salads and baked potatoes. For variety, add onions or 2 ounces of blue cheese. (Blue cheese will add about 40 milligrams of sodium to each tablespoonful of this dressing.)

About 12 calories per tablespoon, or 22 calories per tablespoon when blue cheese is added.

NO-CAL SALAD DRESSING

½ cup of wine vinegar
½ teaspoon of Herb Salt
(see p. 97)
1 tablespoon of fresh
chopped parsley

1 clove of garlic, crushed, or
or ¼ teaspoon of garlic
powder

Mix well. Use other herbs and vinegars for variety. Tarragon is one of the best herbs for salad dressings. And, if available, try the fruit vinegars (they are excellent) such as raspberry or strawberry. You may add ¼ to ½ cup of water to this dressing if it is too vinegary for your taste.

LO-CAL SALAD DRESSING

¼ cup of fine olive oil
¼ cup of water
¼ cup of wine or fruit
vinegar

1 clove of garlic, crushed
½ teaspoon of salt
1 teaspoon of dried tarragon

Blend by shaking in a jar and letting stand for several hours before its first use. Always shake before using.

Use different herbs for variety.

For extra tang, add 1 teaspoon of Dijon mustard.

About 33 calories per tablespoon. (Don't be concerned about the water in this recipe—it helps spread the flavors and saves calories. Many commercial recipes use water to save calories, just as this one does.)

BALSAMIC NO-CAL DRESSING

¾ cup of water
¼ cup of balsamic vinegar
3 teaspoons of capers
2 teaspoons of prepared
Dijon mustard

1½ teaspoons of dried basil
1 tablespoon of fresh
parsley, chopped
(optional)

Blend at high speed. (Adjust vinegar to taste.)

About 2 calories per tablespoon.

Meats: Beef, Pork, and Veal

You probably have some favorite ways of preparing meat, and you should feel free to use them if the recipes call for lean cuts and no added fat or oil.

Here are three quick ways of flavoring steak or lean beef patties. Similar seasonings can be used with other cuts of beef.

STEAK AND HAMBURGER TERIYAKI STYLE

Sprinkle a 4-ounce (raw weight) lean beef patty with ground ginger, freshly ground pepper, just a touch of garlic powder and onion powder, and a teaspoon of soy sauce. Try a low-salt variety of soy sauce if you wish to be more moderate in your salt intake. My favorite brand is Tamari. Pan- or oven-broil without added fat. (A 4-ounce patty reduces to 3 ounces during cooking.)

Use the same seasonings with steak, calculating your portion size as directed three paragraphs below.

Variation 1. Italian Seasonings. Sprinkle liberally with garlic powder and onion powder, and your choice of herbs such as oregano, basil, thyme, marjoram, and parsley. Add a touch of freshly ground black pepper. This recipe doesn't need salt, so don't add any until you serve the hamburger and taste it. After turning in the pan, spread hamburger with a teaspoon of catsup or chili sauce.

Variation 2. Chili Seasonings. Sprinkle liberally with Mexican chili powder, paprika, and a dash of cayenne pepper. Cumin and basil will make interesting additions to the flavor as well. Add salt after tasting at the table.

Lean beef and extra-lean hamburger will average about 55 calories per cooked ounce. Serving size is 3 ounces cooked (165 calories) on the 600/900-calorie rotations, 4½ ounces cooked (248 calories) on the 1200-calorie rotation, and 6 ounces cooked (330 calories) at the higher levels.

STEAK FLAMED IN BRANDY

Flavor your steak with your favorite seasonings and pan-broil.
Just before serving, pour 1 ounce of brandy over the steak and
light fumes with a match. Let it burn out before serving.

Just about all of the calories in the brandy burn off, so
figure about 55 calories an ounce for lean meat.

MARINATED FLANK STEAK

You can use either of the following two marinades with any cut
of steak, but I like to use flank steak because it is one of the
leanest cuts of meat and the marinade tenderizes it. In addition,
the use of either marinade is excellent for outdoor grilling. If you
use any other cut of steak, be sure to trim all the visible fat (most
of the calories in any cut of steak come from fat, *not* protein).

2 pounds of flank steak	1 bay leaf
1 tablespoon of salad oil	2 cloves of garlic, minced
½ cup of dry white wine	2 teaspoons of chopped chives
1 small onion, minced	
¼ teaspoon of thyme leaves	

Steak must be marinated overnight to obtain the full tenderizing
and flavoring effect. Use a covered bowl or two plastic Baggies
(one might leak). (An extra tenderizing and even more flavorful
effect can be obtained if you take the trouble to pierce the steak
with the tines of a fork on both sides, before putting it in the
marinade, at intervals of about a ¼ inch.)

Broil about 4 minutes on each side, basting with marinade
as you turn. Use all of the marinade. Slice thinly on the diagonal
to serve (it's both attractive and easy for the diner to deal with
diagonal cuts), and cover with sauce from the pan. Add salt and
pepper to taste at the table.

Here is an Oriental marinade that will have you salivating
every time you think about it after you have sampled it:

1 tablespoon of salad oil	1-inch cube of fresh ginger,
¼ cup of Tamari	peeled and grated or minced
¼ cup of dry red wine	(it must be fresh ginger—
4 cloves of garlic, minced	the powder just won't give
4 scallions, minced	you the flavor of the fresh
6 whole peppercorns	root)
¼ teaspoon of ground	
coriander	

Marinate overnight and cook as above.

Each 4-ounce serving of cooked flank steak will contain about 220 calories.

Each 2 pounds of steak (raw weight) will yield about 6 servings. The exact number of servings depends upon the size you desire, and you must remember that there is about 25 percent shrinkage from the raw to the cooked state.

———

HERBED PORK

4 lean pork chops, 1 to	½ teaspoon each of rosemary,
1½ inches thick	thyme, tarragon, oregano,
2 tablespoons of Tamari	sage, and basil
1 teaspoon of cornstarch	Salt and freshly ground black
or flour	pepper to taste
1 clove of garlic, minced	

Trim all visible fat. Puncture the chops with the tines of a fork at intervals of about a ¼ inch. Rub well with the cornstarch or flour. Place the Tamari, herbs, garlic, and pepper in a shallow bowl and marinate the chops for at least 2 hours (preferably overnight). Be sure the chops are coated on both sides with the marinade and turn two or three times. This marinade is an excellent tenderizer. (Add a little more Tamari if there is not enough to coat the chops, and leave a bit remaining in the bottom of your marinating bowl.)

Place chops in a skillet with ½ cup of water, cover, and simmer *very gently* for 45 minutes. Do not boil as this will toughen the meat. Remove chops. Pour off and save the liquid. If you have trimmed the meat well there will be very little fat on top of the liquid. Remove any that remains.

Return chops to the pan and brown on both sides. When done, place on warm platter. Return liquid to skillet and heat, tasting occasionally to determine how much salt to add. You can add more water to taste, or perhaps ¼ cup of dry white wine (the alcohol will evaporate, leaving the flavor). It takes about 2 to 3 minutes to make this sauce.

Pour over the chops and serve (you might want to save a bit of the sauce for a baked potato if that is also on the menu).

Lamb chops can be made with a similar marinade. However, lamb chops should be pan-broiled in a skillet, uncovered, without water, for about 7–8 minutes per side. Remove the chops and add either ½ cup of water or a 50/50 mixture of water and dry red wine to the drippings in the skillet and heat to make a sauce.

The lean meat, separated from all visible fat, will contain about 55 calories per ounce, but unless you do a perfect job of trimming, you should figure about 70 calories per ounce, or about 315 calories for a 4½-ounce serving and 420 calories for a 6-ounce serving.

POT ROAST OF BEEF

This particular roast is made with Italian seasonings.

2 pounds of lean roast (top or bottom round, trimmed) or	1 bay leaf
	1 tablespoon of Italian seasonings*
2 pounds of flank steak	1 28-ounce can of tomatoes
4 cloves of garlic, minced	1 15-ounce can of tomato sauce or puree
2 medium onions, sliced	
1 green pepper, sliced	2 teaspoons of soy sauce
4 stalks of celery, cut in 2-inch pieces	Dash of Worcestershire
	Salt and pepper to taste
6 large carrots, cut in 2-inch pieces	Optional: ½ cup of hearty red wine
12 new potatoes	

---

* Use a commercial Italian seasoning, or mix your own from oregano, basil, marjoram, tarragon, and thyme, about ½ teaspoon each, plus ¼ teaspoon of rosemary.

Place meat in a large roasting pan, and cover with minced garlic and slices of onions and green pepper. Place other vegetables and potatoes all around the meat.

Mix the soy sauce and Worcestershire sauce in either the tomatoes or the tomato sauce, and then add both to the roast (together with the wine, if you use it). Add all the other seasonings.

Cook in a slow oven (250 degrees) for 4 to 5 hours, or until meat falls apart when prodded with the tines of a fork.

Makes 6 or 8 servings (3 or 4 ounces of meat, cooked), which, with vegetables, will average 275 or 325 calories per serving, respectively.

VEAL LOAF

1 pound of ground veal	½ cup of dry bread crumbs
1 15-ounce can of tomato kidney beans, drained	1 egg
	2 tablespoons of soy sauce
⅛ teaspoon of cayenne pepper	1 teaspoon of basil
1 15-ounce can of tomato sauce	Dash of Worcestershire sauce
1 teaspoon of oregano	Freshly ground black pepper to taste

Puree beans in a food processor. Remove and add to veal. Blend in bread crumbs, egg, soy sauce, Worcestershire sauce, black and cayenne peppers, and about 3 tablespoons of the tomato sauce.

Place in deep baking dish, cover with remaining sauce, and sprinkle with oregano and basil. If you like your loaves hot, sprinkle with additional cayenne.

Bake 1 hour at 350 degrees.

Makes 8 servings (4 ounces of loaf, plus sauce) at about 220 calories per serving.

Fowl

ALMOND CHICKEN

3 pounds of chicken
breasts, skinned and
boned
⅓ cup of Tamari
1-inch cube of fresh
ginger, finely minced (or
1 teaspoon of dry
ground ginger)
3 cloves of garlic, finely
minced (or 1 teaspoon of
powder)

½ cup of whole-wheat
flour
½ cup of finely ground
almonds
½ teaspoon of salt
½ teaspoon of pepper
2 tablespoons of peanut or
corn oil

In a large bowl, combine the soy sauce, ginger, and garlic. Cut the chicken into bite-size chunks and marinate in the soy mixture while you prepare the other ingredients.

In another bowl, combine flour, almonds, and the rest of the seasonings. Add this to the chicken and toss until the chicken is coated with the flour mixture.

Heat the oil in a wok or large skillet on high heat. When the oil is hot, add the chicken, and turn the heat down to medium. Cook covered, stirring often, about 20 minutes.

This goes well with rice and a green vegetable.

Makes 8 servings at 223 calories per serving, not including the rice and vegetables.

BAKED CHICKEN

There are countless ways to prepare poultry, and I will present several other recipes in addition to the simplest baking recipes later in this book. During the 600/900-calorie rotations of your diet it is probably best to keep the recipes simple, in order to be sure a few hundred extra calories don't sneak into your daily diet. Oven baking is one of those simple but delicious ways to prepare chicken.

Line a baking pan with foil and lay out the pieces of a small fryer. Flavor with your favorite seasonings and bake at 300 degrees for approximately 1 hour. Skin before eating (much of the flavor of the seasonings will have penetrated to the flesh of the chicken during baking; however, add more at the table, if desired).

Try the following different combinations of seasonings for variety.

Variation 1. Sprinkle liberally with onion, garlic powder, and Herb Salt (page 97). Or make your own selection of herbs, using one or more of the following: marjoram, oregano, rosemary, tarragon, or thyme. Add freshly ground black pepper.

Variation 2. Sprinkle liberally with chili powder, paprika, and add a dash of cayenne pepper. Add salt at the table after tasting.

Variation 3. Calories are significantly less if the chicken is skinned *before* baking. But skinning prior to cooking creates a problem since the meat is likely to dry out. You can prevent this by coating the skinned chicken with a basting sauce made from ½ cup of catsup, 2 tablespoons of Tamari, and 2 ounces of sherry. Then sprinkle with other herbs of your choice. (Additional salt is not needed because of the soy sauce.) Cover the chicken lightly with a piece of aluminum foil for about half of the actual cooking time and it will stay moist.

White meat baked without the skin is about 45 calories an ounce, dark meat is about 50. On 600/900 rotations, the serving size is 3 ounces cooked (135 and 150 calories for white and dark meat, respectively). On the 1200-calorie rotation, the serving size is 4½ ounces (208 and 225 calories for white and dark meat, respectively). On 1500- and 1800-calorie rotations, the serving size is 6 ounces (270 and 300 calories for white and dark meat, respectively). Basting sauce will add between 15 and 30 calories per serving, depending on size.

LEMON-BAKED CHICKEN

About 3½ pounds of
  chicken pieces, skinned
¼ cup of lemon juice
1 onion, cut into chunks
1 clove of garlic, finely
  diced

¼ teaspoon of thyme
¼ teaspoon of marjoram
¼ teaspoon of freshly ground
  pepper
1 tablespoon of fresh parsley,
  chopped

Combine all ingredients in a 3-quart casserole dish and marinate for at least an hour, covered in the refrigerator. Stir occasionally.

Bake, covered, in a preheated oven at 350 degrees for 1½ hours.

Serves 4 to 6. See Baked Chicken for the calorie count. (This chicken is so good as a leftover you may wish to double the recipe.)

CHICKEN TOMASI

This dish is adapted from a traditional Hungarian recipe. We are not sure it originated in the town of Tomasi, but we like the name!

3 pounds of chicken pieces, skinned
2 teaspoons of butter
1 medium onion, chopped
1 clove of garlic, minced
5 teaspoons of paprika
¼ teaspoon of cayenne
½ cup of bouillon
1 cup of plain yogurt
¼ cup of low-fat milk
Salt and black pepper to taste

Melt 1 teaspoon of butter in a large saucepan and brown the chicken pieces. Remove the chicken from the pan and drain on paper towels on a platter.

Melt the remaining butter in the pan, and sauté the onion and garlic, covering the saucepan, until the onions are clear.

Place the chicken back in the pan, sprinkle with paprika and cayenne, and pour the bouillon in. Simmer, covered, until the chicken is tender.

Again, remove the chicken from the pan, and remove the pan from the burner. Let the bouillon cool for several minutes. Cooling is essential to prevent the dairy products from curdling.

When the bouillon is lukewarm, stir in the yogurt and the milk until smooth. Replace the skillet over low heat, add salt and pepper to taste, and put the chicken back in.

Reheat until hot—but do not let the sauce boil!

The chicken contains approximately 300 calories for a 6-ounce serving. Add 10 calories for each tablespoon of sauce.

Serves 6 to 8.

Fish

POACHED FISH FILLETS

Poaching is about the simplest low-calorie way to prepare fish fillets as well as fish steaks, such as salmon or halibut.

2 pounds of fish fillets or steaks	Herb Salt to taste (p. 97)
1 cup of dry white wine	Sliced lemon and sprigs of parsley for garnish
2 cups of water	Optional ingredients:
1 tablespoon of chopped fresh parsley	1 onion, thinly sliced
1 bay leaf	1 carrot, thinly sliced
1 lemon, thinly sliced	1 cup of bottled clam juice

Combine wine, water, chopped parsley, bay leaf, thinly sliced lemon, and Herb Salt, plus optional ingredients, and bring to a boil in a saucepan. Reduce heat and simmer for 30 minutes. Strain.

Divide fish into portions of approximately 4 to 8 ounces, depending on what your daily menu calls for (the weight will be reduced by 25 percent during baking). Place in a casserole dish with bouillon. Cover and bake at 300 degrees for about 20 minutes, or until fish flakes when tested with a fork.

Remove fish to a warm platter with a couple of tablespoons of the fish bouillon and cover with foil to keep moist. Place the remainder of the bouillon in the saucepan and heat to reduce by half.

Pour over the fish before serving and garnish with additional lemon slices and parsley.

Shortcut Method: I have had excellent luck with this dish using a shortcut method that takes only about 5 minutes of preparation once you gather the ingredients.

Place your fish in the center of a piece of aluminum foil large enough to fold over the fish. Place the foil and fish in a baking pan. Season with Herb Salt and any of the other ingredients from the above recipe that you like. Cut the liquid ingredients in the above recipe to ½ cup of white wine, ½ cup of water, and (optional) ½ cup of clam juice. Pour directly over the fish and fold the foil tightly to make a perfect seal.

Place in a preheated 300-degree oven and bake for about 30 minutes, or until fish flakes when tested with a fork.

Let the fish cool a bit before serving. Taste the bouillon and reduce, if necessary, to obtain the strength of flavor you prefer. Then pour over the fish before serving.

Fish fillets will average about 50 calories an ounce, cooked. Serving size is 3 ounces cooked on 600/900 rotations, 4½ ounces cooked on 1200, and 6 ounces cooked on higher intakes.

Serves 6 to 8 (depending on where you are in the Rotation Diet).

BAKED FISH FILLETS

1½ pounds of fillets (sole, flounder, etc.)
1 tablespoon of oil
1 tablespoon of lemon juice

2 tablespoons of fresh parsley, chopped
1 lemon (6 wedges)
Salt and freshly ground black pepper to taste

In the bottom of a shallow baking or broiling pan, spread the oil, lemon juice, and pepper. Swish the fish around in the pan, coating both sides. Sprinkle with parsley.

Broil 3–4 minutes on each side or until the edges are browned. Serve with lemon wedges, and add salt to taste at the table.

See Poached Fish Fillets for the calorie counts.

Serves 4 to 6 (depending upon where you are in the Rotation Diet).

BAKED OR BROILED RAINBOW TROUT

4 small trout (about ¾ pound each)
1 tablespoon of oil

Herb Salt to taste (p. 97)
Freshly ground black pepper to taste

Preheat oven to 500 degrees. Pour oil into aluminum-lined baking pan, swish fish around well in the oil, season, and bake for about 12 minutes, or until fish flakes easily with a fork. You may broil if you prefer.

If you like your fish with garlic and onion flavorings, sprinkle with garlic powder and onion powder before baking.

Serves 4. Edible portion, approximately 4 ounces, will contain about 125 calories.

ROYAL INDIAN SALMON

4 salmon steaks, 1 inch thick
¼ cup of chicken or vegetable bouillon
2 tablespoons of lemon juice
½ teaspoon of fennel seeds, crushed
¼ teaspoon of cumin
¼ teaspoon of ground coriander
Dash of salt
Freshly ground black pepper

Place the steaks in a shallow glass pan. Pour the bouillon and the lemon juice over the steaks. Add the seasonings.

Marinate, covered, in the refrigerator for at least 2 hours, turning the steaks occasionally.

To cook, place the steaks on a foil-covered broiling pan. Spoon 2 teaspoons of the marinade on top of each steak. Place under the broiler for 6 to 8 minutes, or until slightly brown on the edges. Turn steaks over, spoon on the remaining marinade, and broil for an additional 6 to 8 minutes.

A 6-ounce serving will contain approximately 330 calories.

Note: This dish has a delicate, aristocratic flavor—not too spicy or hot in the way many people expect Indian cooking to be.

Pasta

MY FAVORITE PASTA

Garlic and Clam Sauce

This is an unusual but very tasty garlic and clam sauce that combines additional vegetables with the clams so that a large serving can use a bit less spaghetti or linguini, and a little more sauce, with fewer calories per portion.

2 tablespoons of fine olive oil	Dash of cayenne
4 cloves of garlic, minced	2 6- or 7-ounce cans of minced clams
½ cup of chopped onion	½ cup of chopped green peppers
½ pound of mushrooms, sliced	Salt and freshly ground black pepper to taste
1½ teaspoons of dried thyme leaves	
2 tablespoons of chopped fresh parsley	

Sauté the onion, green peppers, and garlic in the olive oil until translucent (add a little water and cover if necessary during this process). Add the mushrooms and continue heating in the covered saucepan for about 3 minutes. Add the remaining ingredients, including all the liquid that comes with the clams, and heat until hot in the covered saucepan.

Makes 4 servings (approximately 70 calories each).

Serve with 1 cup of spaghetti or linguini (2 ounces dry; about 200 calories) and Parmesan cheese (optional).

Total calories per serving are 270. Add 50 calories per tablespoon of Parmesan cheese.

Meat Sauce

1 pound of extra-lean chopped meat	1 stalk of celery, chopped
1 large onion, chopped	1 green pepper, chopped
1 28-ounce can of tomatoes	1 teaspoon of chili powder
1 6-ounce can of tomato paste	½ teaspoon of oregano
1 tablespoon of Worcestershire sauce	½ teaspoon of basil
	Salt and pepper to taste

Brown the first four ingredients (if you have bought extra-lean beef, there will be no fat to pour off). Add the remaining ingredients and bring to a boil. Reduce heat immediately and simmer, uncovered, for about an hour or until sauce reaches desired consistency. You may add a small amount of water to taste, or ¼ cup of dry red wine, during cooking.

Makes 6 servings of about 125 calories each.

Served with 1 cup of cooked spaghetti the total calories are about 325. Add 50 calories per tablespoon of Parmesan cheese, if used.

Vegetables

The best ways to prepare most vegetables to keep the calorie content at a minimum are steamed, boiled in a very small amount of water, or cooked in a microwave, according to its directions. During the 600/900 rotations, we use no fats or other additions that will increase the calories unnecessarily—we concentrate on herbs. At higher intake levels you can dress your vegetables up with small amounts of fat and other caloric additions.

All vegetables can be eaten plain, or with just a sprinkle of salt (or, better, Herb Salt, page 97) and freshly ground pepper, if you desire. The following recipes add a bit of interest—you may not have considered how herbs and spices can turn the ordinary into the exotic. When you use herbs and spices for seasoning you will find it easy to reduce or eliminate both salt and fat in your cooking.

Remember that most vegetables are at their nutritious best

when eaten raw. While I include tasty ways of cooking the vegetables in the Rotation Diet, you will do well to eat one vegetable raw each day. And cooked vegetables are best when served crisp.

ACORN SQUASH

For baking, cut in half lengthwise, spoon out seeds, and bake face down on aluminum foil at 350 degrees for about 45 minutes, or until tender. Season with salt and pepper to taste at the table. Try a sprinkle of cloves, ginger, or nutmeg for variety.

Serves 2 at 56 calories per half of squash.

ASPARAGUS

Caraway Asparagus

If you use fresh asparagus, cut off the tough part of the stalk and cook the spears in a small amount of water for about 12 minutes or until tender. You can also steam asparagus if you prefer, or use your microwave according to directions. The texture of the tips is best preserved by steaming the asparagus standing upright and covered in a deep saucepan. Peel back an inch or so of the outer stalks before placing them in the saucepan. Add about ½ teaspoon of caraway seeds for each cup of asparagus, plus freshly ground black pepper to taste. (Follow directions on the package for frozen asparagus.)

Cold Dijon Asparagus

Mix 1 tablespoon of Dijon mustard with 1 tablespoon of plain yogurt and ¼ teaspoon of tarragon. Spread over chilled asparagus. Add salt and freshly ground black pepper to taste.

Serving size is 1 cup at 18 calories. Add 8 calories for the Dijon dressing.

GREEN BEANS ALMONDINE

1 10-ounce package of
   frozen green beans
¼ cup of water

Dash of salt and pepper
2 tablespoons of slivered
   almonds

Cook green beans in water until crispy tender, add remaining ingredients, and simmer for an additional 5 minutes.

    Makes 4 servings of ½ cup at 38 calories per serving.

GREEN BEANS WITH CHIVES

1 pound of fresh green
   beans (2 10-ounce
   packages frozen)
2 tablespoons of chopped
   fresh parsley

1 tablespoon of chopped
   chives (or scallions)
½ tablespoon of Herb Salt
   (p. 97)

Steam or simmer (in ¼ cup of water) unseasoned beans until tender (or follow directions for your microwave). Sprinkle other ingredients just before serving.

    Variations. Beans can be made with ½ pound of mushrooms, 1 large sliced onion, or 1 can of baby onions, without changing the caloric value of a ½-cup serving to any great extent.

    Makes 8 servings of ½ cup at 18 calories per serving.

GINGERED BEETS

You can use canned baby beets, or cook the beets yourself, leaving on about 1 inch of the stem and root ends. Small beets will take about ½ hour to cook in boiling water. I have not tried to cook them yet in my microwave.

    Drain most of the liquid from the beets, and sprinkle lightly with ground ginger (about ¼ teaspoon per ½ cup) before serving. You can add a couple of tablespoons of cider vinegar if you want some extra zing. Top with a tablespoon of chopped fresh parsley.

Serving size is ½ cup at 29 calories per serving.

BROCCOLI

Broccoli is one of my favorite vegetables. It not only tastes good, but it's a powerhouse when it comes to nutritional value—plenty of vitamins A and C, plus fiber. Broccoli is also a good source of calcium and iron. It should become one of your vegetable staples.

Broccoli is excellent when cooked in the microwave, steamed, or simmered in ¼ cup of water or bouillon until it can be penetrated with the tines of a fork, but is still crisp. If you don't care much for broccoli without a sauce, just sprinkle each serving with a teaspoon of Parmesan cheese and you have the 600/900-calorie rotation version of Broccoli au Gratin.

Serving size is ½ cup at 30 calories per serving; add about 15 calories for the cheese.

BROCCOLI WITH BLACK OLIVES

1 large bunch of broccoli (about 1½ pounds)	4 tablespoons of Parmesan cheese
1 tablespoon of olive oil	Salt and pepper to taste
1 clove of garlic, minced	
2 ounces of pitted black olives	

Cook broccoli in a small amount of water for 10 minutes (or in a microwave according to directions). Drain. Sauté garlic in olive oil until lightly brown. Add broccoli and cook over low heat for 5 minutes (do not overcook). Add olives and heat 2 more minutes. Serve immediately and sprinkle with cheese. Add salt and pepper at the table.

Serves 4 at 90 calories per serving.

CARROTS

In my own diet, carrots run a close second to broccoli as my favorite vegetable. I like carrots sliced and cooked in the microwave with nothing but a bit of water (follow your own microwave recipe). Dill and/or chives make good seasonings.

Carrots a l'Orange

For this variation, add 1 tablespoon of slivered orange peel to each cup of slivered or sliced carrots before cooking. Add Herb Salt (page 97) to taste after serving.

And, of course, in place of the orange, you can use 1 tablespoon of fresh (1 teaspoon of dried) dillweed or 2 tablespoons of chives or chopped scallions for variety.

Serving size is ½ cup at 23 calories per serving.

CARROTS WITH ONIONS

3 cups of carrots, sliced   Salt, pepper, and fresh
1 onion, chopped   parsley to taste
¼ cup of water

Place ingredients in saucepan, bring to a boil, and then simmer gently until cooked.

Makes 6 servings at 27 calories per serving.

BRAISED CARROTS AND CELERY

The word "braise" refers to a method of cooking in fat, with very little moisture. Naturally, when it comes to weight management, the worst thing you can do in preparing meals is to use even a drop more fat than you need for flavoring. My "braising" is done in the microwave, or in a small amount of water on top of the stove.

For each serving:

1 carrot, in ¼-inch slices
1 stalk of celery, in 2-inch slices

Place in saucepot with ¼ cup of water (¼ cup of water regardless of number of carrots and celery, up to a maximum of four carrots or stalks) and simmer until crisp, but definitely not soft.

Pour off water and mix with 1 tablespoon of butter for all of the 4 servings (a little less than 1 teaspoon per serving).

When using a microwave, follow the directions that come with your oven, and add a small amount of butter after cooking.

Chives are about the best accompaniment that I know of with carrots and celery. Add about ¼ teaspoon of chives per serving, before cooking, if you like.

About 25 calories per serving.

SAVORY STEAMED CAULIFLOWERETS

Cut up a medium head of cauliflower into 2-inch flowerets, and, for each cup of cauliflower, sprinkle with ½ teaspoon of oregano and ½ teaspoon of savory. Steam until tender.

Serving size is 1 cup at 30 calories per serving.

OLD THYMEY PEAS

Maybe you remember the old folk song Simon and Garfunkel made famous in the sixties: *Scarborough Fair.* Here's a recipe that uses all the lovely herbs mentioned in that song.

1 package (10½ ounces) of frozen peas, or 1½ cups fresh
1 teaspoon of parsley

½ teaspoon of sage
½ teaspoon of rosemary
½ teaspoon of thyme

Cook peas in ¼ cup of water until barely tender. Add seasonings and cook 1 minute more before serving.

Variations: Peas go well with a squeeze of lemon and a pinch of basil (about ⅙ of a lemon and ½ teaspoon of basil per ½ cup). Add salt and pepper to taste.

Serving size for either recipe is ½ cup at 57 calories per serving.

PEAS AND BABY ONIONS

1 package (10½ ounces) of frozen peas, or 1½ cups fresh
1 small can of baby onions, or 1 large onion, sliced

1 tablespoon of butter
Herb Salt (p. 97)
Freshly ground black pepper to taste

Fresh onions should be sautéed in butter until translucent. Add peas and ¼ cup of water. Cook until tender.

If using canned onions, cooks peas first until tender; add onions and butter, and warm.

This is a traditional dish with baked or poached fish. It is especially complementary to salmon.

Makes 4 servings of ½ cup at 75 calories per serving.

BROWN OR WILD RICE

2 cups of brown or wild rice
1 tablespoon of butter or oil
4 cups of bouillon (meat or vegetable)

Other seasonings to taste— for example, 1 tablespoon of chopped chives, scallions, or Herb Salt (p. 97), depending on the bouillon

Melt butter in saucepan, add rice, and stir until rice is coated. Add bouillon, cover and bring to boil. Reduce heat and simmer gently for 45 minutes, or until all of the liquid has been absorbed.

The rice will expand to 4 cups in volume and provide 8 ½-cup servings, which, prepared in this way, will contain about 105 calories each.

SPINACH AND BROCCOLI CASSEROLE

2 10-ounce packages of frozen spinach (chopped)
1 10-ounce package of frozen broccoli (chopped)
½ cup of water
1 can of mushroom soup
½ cup of seasoned bread crumbs
½ cup of grated Parmesan cheese
½ cup of grated cheddar cheese
1 teaspoon each of garlic and onion powder
½ cup of low-fat milk
Salt and pepper to taste

Cook broccoli and spinach in water until completely thawed (but not cooked). Stir in remaining ingredients, place in large casserole dish, and cover with seasoned bread crumbs. Bake at 350 degrees for 35–40 minutes.

Makes about 12 servings of ½ cup at approximately 85 calories per serving.

This is an excellent dish as a main course. Just double or triple the serving size, and calculate the calories appropriately.

STIR-FRY SPINACH (OR OTHER GREENS)

1 pound of fresh spinach (or other greens)
1 tablespoon of oil (olive oil preferred)
1 medium onion, sliced thin
Herb Salt to taste (p. 97)
Freshly ground black pepper to taste

Wash and drain greens. Heat oil in skillet and sauté onions for 1 minute. Add greens and stir until leaves are wilted and greens are hot—about 1 minute more on medium heat.

Serve with a squeeze of lemon or a sprinkle of grated cheese.

Makes 4 servings at about 60 calories per serving.

BAKED TOMATO

2 fresh tomatoes
1 clove of garlic, minced
¼ teaspoon of tarragon
¼ teaspoon of basil

1 tablespoon of Parmesan cheese
Freshly ground black pepper taste

Slice tomatoes in half. Place in shallow baking pan, flat side up. Combine seasonings and cheese, and sprinkle over tomatoes. Bake at 350 degrees for about 30 minutes, or until tender.

Makes 4 servings at about 28 calories per serving.

STIR-FRY VEGETABLES

If you are already experienced in stir-frying, do your vegetables in the way you like them (as long as you keep the fat content down).

This is actually a method of skillet frying that comes close to duplicating the results obtained with a wok.

1 thinly sliced green pepper
4 large carrots (½-inch pieces)
2 medium onions, thinly sliced
3 cloves of garlic, chopped
4 stalks of celery (2-inch pieces)

1 tablespoon of butter or oil
½ cup of chopped cabbage
1 pound of fresh greens
2 tablespoons of soy sauce
Freshly ground black pepper
Pinch of marjoram and thyme

Melt butter in skillet on low heat as you begin to slice your vegetables. I add to the skillet, as I slice them, green pepper, carrots, onions, garlic, and celery, in that order, stirring occasionally. Increase heat to medium for 2 to 3 minutes, then add cabbage and greens, and marjoram and thyme. Cook on medium to medium-high heat, stirring almost continuously, until greens have wilted but other vegetables are still crisp. Add soy sauce and pepper to taste.

Serve with Brown or Wild Rice (page 94), which you will

have started about 1 hour before the stir-fry, and 2 tablespoons of grated cheese.

Serves four, with each serving containing about 110 calories. Add about 90 calories for each half cup of plain cooked brown rice and 100 calories for the cheese. Add additional calories if rice is cooked with any added fat.

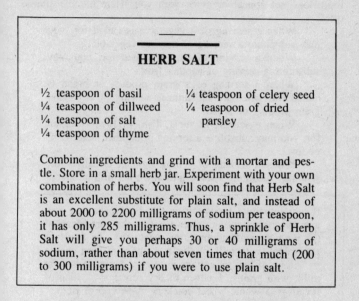

HERB SALT

½ teaspoon of basil
¼ teaspoon of dillweed
¼ teaspoon of salt
¼ teaspoon of thyme

¼ teaspoon of celery seed
¼ teaspoon of dried parsley

Combine ingredients and grind with a mortar and pestle. Store in a small herb jar. Experiment with your own combination of herbs. You will soon find that Herb Salt is an excellent substitute for plain salt, and instead of about 2000 to 2200 milligrams of sodium per teaspoon, it has only 285 milligrams. Thus, a sprinkle of Herb Salt will give you perhaps 30 or 40 milligrams of sodium, rather than about seven times that much (200 to 300 milligrams) if you were to use plain salt.

PERMISSIBLE SUBSTITUTIONS AND OTHER ALTERATIONS TO THE ROTATION DIET

Substitutions

The daily menus for the Rotation Diet have been developed to provide maximum nutritional value at all caloric levels. That's why it's best to stick with them as closely as possible. In addition, my experience in reviewing thousands of eating diaries indicates that deviations are likely to lead to increased calories, and increased calories will tend to slow your weight loss. The reason for the impact of deviations is usually quite simple to understand: most of us tend to prefer the foods that have more calories (have more fat or are sweeter) in any given food category!

Nevertheless, you can make substitutions if any particular food does not appeal or agree with you. Here are the simple rules:

When a serving of a vegetable is called for, you may substitute a serving of another vegetable.

When a serving of fruit is called for, you may substitute a serving of another fruit.

When a serving of a grain product or bread is called for, you may substitute a serving of any other grain product or bread.

When a serving of meat, fish, or fowl is called for, you may substitute a serving of another meat, fish, or fowl.

When a serving of a milk product is called for, you may substitute a serving of any other milk product.

If you substitute foods during the diet, make sure you use the correct serving sizes whether they are identical (as with vegetables, fruit, or meat, fish, or fowl) or equivalent (with milk products, 1 ounce of hard cheese = ½ cup of low-fat cottage cheese = 1 cup of low-fat milk; with grains, 1 ounce of dry cereal = 1 slice of bread = 5 whole-wheat crackers = ½ cup of rice).

You should remember however, that your nutritional needs are best served by a wide variety of foods. In addition, there is another potential value to a wide variety of foods: variety in your choices of foods will ensure that you do not take in particularly large amounts of any given preservative or whatever pesticides are used in growing a particular food product.

I could be picky-picky about which substitutions are most closely equivalent in calories, but I don't think it is worth your effort to be concerned about 5 or 10 calories, more or less. And as for other nutritional values, you will do best if you choose foods that are similar to each other as substitutions. For example, one variety of green vegetable for another, one variety of winter squash for another, and so forth. In either case, you will not do much damage, provided you stick to the wide-variety principle, and do not continually eat just one or two foods from a given category.

Study the menus, and the recipes, and you will soon learn serving sizes if you don't already know them.

Skipping Meals, Combining Meals, Reversing the Order of Meals

Do you have to follow the menus exactly? Or can you eat breakfast for dinner and vice versa?

We have many people in the Vanderbilt Weight Management Program who juggle the foods around in the day to please themselves and it seems to work out very well. But, in order to be sure that you are obtaining adequate nutrition, *be sure that you end up eating what I suggest in each day's menu.* Make any substitutions from the appropriate categories. Sometimes changes of this kind do interfere with weight loss, especially if you end up eating everything at night (or at the end of whatever is your workday, before you go to sleep).

If you have unusual hours, try eating the meals in the order that they fit into your workday (breakfast first, etc.), and then make alterations to please yourself if this doesn't turn out to be satisfactory.

Most alterations in the daily eating patterns will not make a great deal of difference. During the 600-calorie rotations, just have two servings of a grain product, two servings of a milk product, two different vegetables, two different fruits, and about 3 ounces of lean meat, fish, or fowl—and that's about as simple as I can make it!

During the 900-calorie rotations, add another grain product and another serving of lean meat, fish, or fowl. There is also room for 1 teaspoon of fat or oil for seasoning or spread.

During the 1200-calorie rotation, make it a total of four grains, two milk products, two different fruits and two different vegetables, and two servings of lean meat, fish, or fowl. And you also have room for 1 tablespoon of fat or oil for seasoning or spread.

Vegetarian Substitutions

Vegetarians can use the Rotation Diet by substituting a complementary protein dish composed of combinations of legumes, grains, seeds, and nuts for meat, fish, or fowl. A combination of a grain with a legume will provide the most complete protein with the fewest calories. A soy product such as tofu may also be substituted any time a food of animal origin is called for in the menus. Adding a small amount of cheese to plant foods will increase the quality of the available protein. A half cup of beans with a half cup of rice will approximate the caloric value of a 3-ounce serving of lean meat (cooked).

DIET DRINKS
(AND THOSE WITH SUGAR)

I hope there is one thing that I can persuade you to do during the Rotation Diet, and that is to give up drinking diet drinks for the entire three weeks. I want you to see for yourself whether using diet drinks is keeping alive your taste for sweets, and ultimately leading you to overeat on sweets that do contain calories.

I would be willing to bet that diet sweeteners are keeping alive your yen for sweets and leading you to overeat. In fact, I'll give you odds because I have never yet met a person who is completely satisfied with the use of artificial sweeteners and who doesn't periodically overindulge on "the real thing" in a way that is disastrous for weight control.

If I can persuade you to give up diet drinks, and if you are at all like participants in the Vanderbilt Weight Management Program, you will soon notice an increase in your taste sensitivity.

The use of diet drinks may be deadening your sensitivity to sweetness, leading you to require more than the normal amount of sweetness to satisfy your palate. If this has happened to you, and you decide to give up the use of artificial sweeteners, in a matter of just one or two weeks natural, unsweetened foods will begin to taste unbelievably sweet, and it will become much easier for you to stick with your diet or to increase your intake of more nutritious foods.

In my opinion, diet drinks (and artificially sweetened desserts) just turn on your appetite without satisfying it, possibly leading you to overeat at other times. When you need a drink, try water! If you crave something sweet, use your *safe fruit*. If you are thirsty and crave something sweet, do both—eat your fruit and have a drink of water.

The food processors who manufacture diet foods are capitalizing on the human preference for sweetness in food, and they may have you "hooked"! Try quitting the use of diet preparations, and the difficulty you experience will prove my point.

Think about it for a few moments. Somebody "out there" is making a fortune feeding you artificial diet sweeteners, products with no nutritional value, and you are gulping them down and staying fat!

If cutting out the use of all artificial sweeteners proves to be difficult, I hope it will make you really angry at the way you are being manipulated for someone else's profit—angry enough at the fact that you've been "hooked"—to perservere in your efforts never to use an artificial sweetener again for the rest of your life.

Cutting out the use of all artificial sweeteners may turn out to be the crucial factor in your efforts to control your weight.

I am a pretty good example of how you can change in your preference for sweets. In contrast with the situation twenty-two years ago, today I use no artificial sweeteners, and, for that matter, I add no sugar to any beverage. I use only small amounts of sugar in baking, usually half or less than what is called for in the usual recipe. (Don't worry about the change in bulk when you do this—I have never found it necessary to make compensatory alterations in the other ingredients.) Compared with my taste for sweets when I was a fat man, my sensitivity to sweetness has increased to the point that most cereals, for example, even Grape-Nuts, taste too sweet to me even without added sugar. Dried fruits such as raisins and dates are at the limit of my tolerance for sweetness. And, whereas half a pound of chocolate might have constituted a binge twenty-two years ago, two bars of candy—perhaps 2 ounces or a quarter of what I might have downed as a fat man—prove to be a perfectly satisfying binge today. It's now possible for me to enjoy a single bar of candy without turning on an insatiable yearning.

While I would much rather see you learn to use small amounts of sugar, honey, or molasses (rather than an artificial sweetener) whenever a sweetener is called for in baking or cooking, I am not rigid in this respect, provided the sweetener is blended with other foods and used in *small* amounts so as not to make the sweetness too intense.

How to Use Sugar

Don't use any drinks that contain "straight sugar," that is, soft drinks. Sugar must be blended as a minor ingredient in the overall recipe for any food.

While white table sugar (sucrose) is found naturally in many foods, it has only been freely available *in its processed form* for about a hundred years.

Considering that about two million years have been involved in the evolution of the human capacity to deal with foods as they are found in our natural environments, it is safe to say that your body is not designed to deal with sugar "straight," which, after all, is a relatively new product. In some persons, processed foods that are high in sucrose set off reactions that are not only terrible for controlling your weight, but lead to what is called "insulin overshoot." Too much insulin will deplete your blood of circulating sugar (glycogen), leading to temporary symptoms of hypoglycemia, or low blood sugar. Although the disease *hypoglycemia* is rare, the temporary symptoms of low blood sugar in normal persons may lead to an increase in appetite. You should avoid using sugar straight, just as you should avoid using an artificial sweetener except as a minor ingredient in a recipe containing other ingredients.

Should you make an effort to give up completely using sugar or eating candy, cakes, and pies?

I don't think so.

An effort to be completely abstinent may build up such a tremendous hidden hunger drive that the slightest deviation can end up in a monstrous binge. In Chapters 9 through 11, I will show you how you can learn to be moderate in your eating habits, and how you can gain control over the tendency to binge on high-calorie foods. There is a happy medium in eating the foods you like best. You must build them into your diet intentionally. Planning to enjoy them, without the driven quality that often accompanies your eating of foods that you feel guilty about enjoying, may actually protect you against a binge.

Some successful people who have been through the Vanderbilt

Program build one to two servings of a rich dessert or candy into their daily maintenance diets. They are now active enough to prevent regaining any weight. I prefer to eat more nutritious foods. I have found my happy medium by including a rich dessert, or possibly some candy, just once a week, or sometimes twice. In this way, I never feel that I am denying myself. However, by not eating such foods every day, I no longer have any yearning for them as a regular part of my diet.

I also make sure that the temptation to eat candy and desserts is not triggered by keeping such foods in the house on a regular basis. Instead, we have bowls of fruit on display and can eat whenever we feel inclined without worrying about the effects on our weight.

What Should You Do if You Are Forced to Deviate from the Diet?

Suppose you are ill and cannot eat the food that is recommended on a particular day's menu? Or, suppose you are out to dinner and end up deviating from the diet because there is nothing available for making appropriate substitutions? How can you get back on the program with the least damage to your weight-loss efforts?

The best way is to go forward to the next day of the Rotation Diet as if nothing happened. Complete the twenty-one days in twenty-one days in spite of any deviations on any given day. Do not lock yourself into a frustrating cycle of starting all over again from Day 1 or attempting to repeat a day's menu over and over again until you get it right. In addition to being frustrating this would work against the nutritional value of the total dietary plan.

No matter what happens, finish the twenty-one days in twenty-one days by going forward on the Rotation Diet; take a break, and you will do better on your second rotation.

THE NUTRITIONAL VALUE OF
THE ROTATION DIET

The Rotation Diet has been designed to approximate the Recommended Dietary Allowances of known major vitamins and minerals over the entire twenty-one-day period that you will use it. The same is true of the suggestions I will make for your maintenance diet.

At the level of 1200 calories and above (including my recommendations for your maintenance diet), the proportions of calories from carbohydrate, fat, and protein are designed to meet the recommendations of the Senate Select Committee on Nutrition and Human Needs: 55 to 60 percent from carbohydrate, 25 to 30 percent from fat, and 15 percent from protein.

Crackpot claims to the contrary, there is no known diet that is more beneficial to your health than the recommendations of the Senate Select Committee on Nutrition and Human Needs.

When calories are reduced below 1200, such as on the 600/900-calorie rotations, the relative percentage from protein increases to around 40 percent, fat decreases to about 20 percent, and carbohydrate decreases to 40 percent. These changes are necessary on a temporary basis since it is important to include enough protein to make the diet palatable, maintain the body's store of protein, and prevent the loss of your muscle tissue.

In spite of the nutritional value of the Rotation Diet, it may be important for you to use a multiple vitamin and mineral supplement while you are on the diet.

Substitutions during the diet may change your intake of certain nutrients. For example, if you do not include milk in your diet, and do not like sardines and salmon from a can, but instead substitute cottage cheese or some other cheese as a calcium source, you will be relatively low on calcium. Although this is not likely to be dangerous on a temporary basis, it might be in the long run. If you do not take in enough calcium to provide for your daily needs, your body leeches it from your bones, gradually weakening them. Then, when you reach a more advanced age, you may be more susceptible to osteoporosis than you would have been with an adequate intake. Thus, I think it would be wise to include a calcium supplement in the form of calcium gluconate, calcium lactate, or calcium carbonate. The last form—

calcium carbonate—can be obtained easily and cheaply by eating one Tums tablet each day. Each Tums tablet supplies 200 milligrams of calcium, which, together with the other sources of calcium in the daily menus, will easily bring your intake up to the RDAs for this nutrient.

There are two other reasons you may need temporary vitamin supplements. First, if you don't care for red meat, you may end up low in some of the B vitamins and iron, since red meat tends to be a major source of these nutrients in most American diets. Substitutions of other meat products or vegetables may not be as rich and lack of these nutrients could leave you feeling weak and lethargic.

Second, while on a reduced-calorie diet, the body's need for vitamins and minerals may change. Although there is no evidence for this effect that I know of, dieting does stress the body, and your need for stress-related vitamins—the B-complex vitamins and vitamin C—may increase. Furthermore, recent research indicates that vigorous exercise may change one's needs for certain B vitamins and iron, and this may occur for you as you change from a sedentary to an active person. A multiple vitamin and mineral tablet will help take care of all of these possibilities.

What brand of vitamin and mineral supplement is best? I recommend that you visit your drugstore and choose the house brand of a multiple vitamin and mineral tablet that contains, in general, amounts that approximate the Recommended Dietary Allowances (RDAs) of the major vitamins and minerals. I would not get anything with higher dosages because too much of certain nutrients may also be bad for you, and your diet, with the permissible substitutions, will provide most, if not all, of them—even at the 600/900-calorie rotations. The store brand of a vitamin and mineral supplement is likely to cost about 5 cents per tablet (versus up to 25 cents for specialty brands that are no better in terms of their nutritional contents).

Discuss supplementing your diet with your physician or nutritionist, and get your druggist's help in choosing the appropriate tablet. And don't be concerned if a few of the nutrients are not exactly at the 100 percent level of the RDAs in the information provided on the label. *Just be sure that you avoid megadoses* and ask the druggist to guide you in the choice of supplement if you are uncertain.

SHOPPING LIST FOR WOMEN'S MENUS OF THE ROTATION DIET

Here is a shopping list to make it easy for you to buy exactly what you will need for the Rotation Diet. I am not entering quantities for you; enter your own in the space provided in case you want to buy enough for the family, or for another person who is going on the Rotation Diet with you. Look at the Week 1 menus, decide upon any substitutions, and add them to this list.

In addition, it is a good idea to check the recipes that are suggested for each day in case you happen to be out of any of the items you will need for cooking.

Week 1 and Week 3

FRUIT
Grapefruit _____
Apples _____
Bananas _____
Berries (in season) _____
Cantaloupe _____
Other (for *safe fruit*) _____
_____

GRAINS
Whole-wheat bread _____
Whole-wheat crackers
(low salt) _____
Breakfast cereal _____
_____
_____

DAIRY PRODUCTS
Milk (skim or low-fat) _____
_____
Cottage cheese (low-fat) _____
Hard cheese _____

MISCELLANEOUS
Mayonnaise (optional) _____
_____
No-cal or lo-cal dressing _____
_____

No-cal beverages (tea, coffee, herb
tea, etc.) _____
_____
Eggs _____
Peanut butter _____

VEGETABLES
Free vegetables: check choice of
Asparagus _____
Celery _____
Chicory _____
Chinese cabbage _____
Cucumbers _____
Endive _____
Escarole _____
Lettuce _____
Parsley _____
Radishes _____
Spinach _____
Watercress _____
Zucchini _____

Other vegetables:
Cauliflower _____
Beets _____
Broccoli _____
Carrots _____
Green beans _____

Asparagus (if not checked above) __   Beefsteak and/or hamburger _____
Green peas _____

HERBS AND SPICES
_____
MEAT, FISH, FOWL   _____
Chicken _____
Fish fillets _____
Tuna (canned) _____   OTHER (for food preparation)
Salmon (canned) _____   _____
Sardines (optional) _____   _____

Week 2

FRUIT   Black olives _____
Grapefruit _____   Chives _____
Apples _____   _____
Bananas _____   No-cal or lo-cal dressing _____
Berries (in season) _____
Cantaloupe _____
Pears (optional) _____   No-cal beverages (tea, coffee, herb
Fresh pineapple (optional) _____   tea, etc.) _____
Raisins _____   _____
Other (for *safe fruit*,   _____
   fruit salad) _____   Eggs _____
_____   Peanut butter _____
_____   Almonds, slivered _____

GRAINS   VEGETABLES
Whole-wheat bread _____   *Free vegetables:* check choice of
Whole-wheat crackers   Asparagus _____
   (low salt) _____   Celery _____
Breakfast cereal (including   Chicory _____
   oatmeal) _____   Chinese cabbage _____
_____   Cucumbers _____
Brown (or wild) rice _____   Endive _____
Pasta _____   Escarole _____
                                        Lettuce _____
DAIRY PRODUCTS   Parsley _____
Milk (skim or low-fat) _____   Radishes _____
_____   Spinach _____
Cottage cheese _____   Watercress _____
Hard cheese _____   Zucchini _____
Parmesan _____
Yogurt (for Chicken Tomasi) _____   *Other vegetables:*
                                        Spinach (if not checked above) __
MISCELLANEOUS   Celery (if not checked above) __
Mayonnaise (optional) _____   Potatoes _____
_____   Baby onions _____

Mushrooms _____
Acorn squash _____
Broccoli _____
Carrots _____
Green beans _____
Tomatoes _____
Green peas _____
Green peppers _____
(Other for stir-fry) _____
_____
_____
_____

Dark kidney beans (for Mexican Bean
    Spread) _____

MEAT, FISH, FOWL
Chicken _____

Fish fillets _____
Tuna (canned) _____
Salmon (canned, optional) ___
Sardines (optional) _____
Canned clams, or chopped meat (for
    pasta sauce) _____
_____
Beefsteak _____
Beef for pot roast (round, flank) __
Salmon steaks _____
Pork chops _____

HERBS AND SPICES
_____
_____
_____

SHOPPING LIST FOR MEN'S MENUS

For all three weeks of the Rotation Diet men should use the shopping list of Week 2 for women as their basic list, and check the daily menus to determine what, if any, substitutions they are going to make. There are only a few meals that will require any changes or additions to the basic shopping list of Week 2 for women. These include Veal Loaf on Day 12 and a suggestion for Baked Trout on Day 14.

7

The Rotation Diet
Activity Plan

As they say, let's call a spade a spade.

I know that if anything is likely to put people off about a weight-management program, it's the suggestion that they need to get physically active. That's why the big money-making commercial weight-loss plans tend to play down the need for physical activity. The advertisers for these programs know that it is difficult for an overweight person to enjoy physical activity. I have one of the advertisements from a major commercial program on my desk right now. You may have seen it, and many others just like it. It reads: "Lose weight easily, without uncomfortable physical activity." If these large commercial programs put the emphasis on physical activity that is truly needed for permanent weight management, many people would not buy their programs.

But I know both the absolute necessity for physical activity in weight management as well as how you feel about it at this time.

Talk about what it feels like! When I was a fat child and a fat man, I felt like a klutz. I didn't walk, I waddled. I was embarrassed to try anything physical because I was convinced that I would be awkward and lousy at it. If I so much as walked on a curb along the street when I was a kid, my mom used to scream, "Watch out, Dick! You'll fall off." (Dick is my nickname.)

Throughout my entire life I avoided gymnasiums. I certainly did not want to let anyone look at all my fat in its naked form. And, up until I was thirty-five years old, there was no way that anyone could convince me that it could possibly *feel good* to be physically active.

I assure you that you can do away with all of these negative feelings about being physical. Follow my advice and I can also assure you that *nothing* will ever make you *feel* thin in the way that being an active person does. If you are at all like me, losing weight by itself does not make you feel like a thin person. No matter what the mirror says, there is still a sense of being fat. All of this changes when you become an *active* thin person.

To begin with, you may feel an increase in your motivation to become more active if you face the facts: if you are a sedentary person, it will be almost impossible for you to manage your weight without finding some way to increase your activity level to the point that nature intended.

Up until the invention of the automobile, and the availability of electricity in our homes and places of work, the average person had to walk seven or eight miles each day. And those people who didn't have to walk quite that much still ended up expending just as much energy because their work required standing, moving around, and a lot more muscle! For the first few million years of our existence as a distinct species of animal, up until about a hundred years ago, human beings had to burn up about 500 calories more energy each day in our work, in maintaining our homes (chopping wood, shoveling coal), and in obtaining food, since there was no electric refrigeration. Our bodies were designed for a high level of physical activity, and our appetites are matched to that level of activity. Because of the nature of life in previous times, we used to be able to eat about 500 calories more each day a hundred years ago, and we were not as likely to get as fat as we are today because we had to burn up all of those extra calories working to stay alive.

Although the need for energy expenditure has decreased significantly in our technologically advanced society, our appetite for food has not. In fact, there is a tendency for inactive persons to eat more than moderately active persons. This may occur, perhaps, out of boredom or as a result of tensions that would normally be lowered through physical activity.

Physical activity is a great regulator of appetite. When sedentary persons get active, they actually tend to eat less than before. Then, as activity levels increase, food intake seems to increase only to the extent that it matches output.

In addition, as long as you remain an active person, Mother Nature puts a special fat-burning mechanism to work to help you stay thin. If you happen to overeat, but get immediately active without missing a day, your body will rev up even higher than it normally does in physical activity, as though it were trying to help you burn off the extra calories you ate the day before. Nature appears to be working to help you stay thin in order to be better at whatever physical thing you ask yourself to do. But consistent physical activity is required. The mechanism will not work as well if your activity becomes sporadic.

SOME ACTIVITIES ARE BETTER THAN OTHERS FOR WEIGHT CONTROL

When it comes to controlling your weight, you get the biggest payoff when you engage in any physical activity that requires you to move your whole body through space.

Just taking a brisk walk burns about twice the calories that you burn doing calisthenics. While swinging your arms and lifting your legs feels like hard work, when you move your whole body through space you move your entire body weight. Moving your whole body feels easier than those arm swings because your body was built for walking. Walking uses your largest muscles (in the buttocks and thighs), and these muscles are placed in the middle of your body. This placement makes for very efficient movement. In contrast, arm swings use smaller muscles and the weight that is being moved extends outward from the moving muscles. That makes for inefficient movement, which is experienced as being harder and is more tiring, in spite of the fact that it burns far fewer calories.

So, the first principle of the Rotation Diet activity program is: move your whole body through space to get the most calorie-burning benefit for every minute that you engage in physical activity.

This principle makes it easy to see what activities are best for weight management: walking, swimming, and gentle jogging (when you get down to desirable weight). These are followed by bicycling (because it also uses the major large muscles in the thighs and buttocks), bouncing on a minitrampoline, and exercises that may move your whole body up and down, but generally in one place rather than through space. Thus, most aerobic dance routines do not give you quite the weight-management benefits of a brisk walk.

Racquet sports can be an excellent route to weight control, provided you learn to play at an advanced level and spend more of your time moving around than standing still and socializing. As you know, tennis was my daily sport for many years, until I discovered the joys of jogging. Racquetball is easier to learn than tennis, and you will tend to burn more calories at racquetball than at tennis in any given period of exercise time.

Rowing—usually on the machines found in many gyms and exercise studios—has recently become a popular weight-management and conditioning activity. It works in spite of your not having to move your whole body through space because it uses so many of the muscle groups throughout your entire body. Rowing can be a valuable activity for persons who cannot do weight-bearing exercise, such as walking, because of injury to their legs or leg joints. However, if you have back problems, discuss the benefits and risks of rowing with your physician, and be sure to start slowly against little resistance until you see how it feels.

YOUR OVERALL ACTIVITY GOAL

Your activity goal is to burn the same number of calories each day that it presently takes to keep the extra fat you now have on your body alive and well!

Let me put it another way: once you have lost your excess weight, your goal is to burn enough calories each day in physical activity to equal the number of calories it used to take to support the extra fat you previously had on your body when you were heavier and inactive.

Because I know the facts from both personal and professional experience, there is little that annoys me more than the claim, made by many commercial weight-control experts who have packaged foods and powders to sell, that diet is more important in weight control than exercise. You probably have heard the statement that "It takes thirty-five miles of walking to lose a pound of fat." Weight-control experts who remind you of this fact then go on to extoll the virtues of their particular diet.

I have no argument about the virtues of diet versus exercise when it comes to *losing weight*. Simply put, diet wins. That's why I have worked to develop the Rotation Diet. But this completely misses the point about the value of physical activity.

The real question is, "What amount of physical activity will it take to keep you at your desired weight, once you have lost all the weight you want to lose?"

Here are the important facts:

It takes about forty-five minutes a day of brisk whole-body activity to equal the number of calories it used to take to support approximately 40 to 50 pounds of extra fat on a sedentary, fat body!

It takes about an hour a day of brisk whole-body physical activity to equal the number of calories it used to take to maintain approximately 60 to 75 pounds of fat on a sedentary, fat body!

(I cannot be more exact then these approximations because of individual differences in metabolic rates.)

Yes, it may take thirty-five miles of walking to lose a pound, but just forty-five minutes of extra walking each day (or a similar amount of time in some other brisk whole-body movement) will keep between 40 and 50 pounds of fat from ever accumulating, or from ever reaccumulating, on your body!

Lose whatever weight you wish to lose with the Rotation Diet. The Rotation Diet will get your weight off just about as fast as any quick-weight-loss diet, without the risks of those diets. As you lose your excess weight, increase your activity level to burn up all the calories that your body formerly used *just to keep its fat alive*. Follow the weekly activity goals that I am about to give you and at the end of just three weeks you will be burning up enough calories to keep 40 to 50 pounds of fat off your body. Then, you may return to your former food intake when you begin your maintenance diet, but you can be confident that you are now active enough *TO PREVENT ALL OF THE FAT YOU HAVE LOST FROM EVER RETURNING*.

YOUR WEEKLY ACTIVITY GOALS

Whatever your level of physical condition, no objective can be more important, and no principle is more fundamental, than this: NEVER HURT YOURSELF.

Competitive athletes may have reasons to exert themselves to the point of injury. The payoff for being a champion may be worth it to them in dollars, even if they end up hobbling around for the rest of their lives. But you and I don't have to go, nor do we need to go, to this extreme in order to control our weight and achieve overall good physical condition. If you hurt yourself, your activity program goes down the tubes. Believe me, once you have become an active person and experienced the joys of being active, if you have to stop you are going to feel terrible! And your feelings will go from terrible to even worse than terrible when you see your weight going up all over again.

As for weekly goals, it is very simple. A beginner in physical activity should aim for:

1. Fifteen minutes a day the first week
2. Gradually increase until you are at thirty minutes a day by the end of the second week
3. Then increase until you reach forty-five minutes a day by the end of the third week

Even though you will not have lost 40 or 50 pounds in three weeks, at the end of this amount of time you will have the security of knowing that, should you need to lose 40 or 50 pounds, you are *already* doing enough in the way of physical activity each day to keep it all off for good. Just use the Rotation Diet one or two times more during the next few months, and you will make it all the way to your desired weight, and you will stay there for good.

The above guidelines for time (forty-five minutes a day) will work when you choose *any* continuous whole-body movement as your activity (walking, bicycling, swimming, jogging). If you choose a racquet sport such as tennis, you need to think more in terms of an hour to an hour and a half, and it needs to be singles tennis, not doubles. Until you become an intermediate to advanced tennis player, you will burn more calories taking a brisk walk than you would in an equal amount of time playing tennis.

Can you take a day off? Yes, if you are tired or feeling under the weather. You should certainly not be active when you have a fever. But extra walking (if nothing else) in a sedentary person's life should become a daily habit.

I will return to more specifics about physical activity later in this chapter.

WHICH ACTIVITY WILL BE BEST FOR YOU?

The next principle of the Rotation Diet activity program is to experiment until you find at least one activity that you really like. It should be something that makes you feel good physically, and that has, in fact, a "moral" impact: you find yourself motivated to continue because you feel like a better person for having done it.

You may find that it is better to have two different activities that you like, rather than one. Not only will this be more interesting, but you are less likely to overdo and injure any particular group of muscles when you alternate activities on a daily basis.

Nothing can be more important, however, than finding some physical activity that becomes a personal expression of your hidden talents and skills. If you take your activity as an "exercise prescription," it will end up feeling like a dose of medicine. Experiment with different activities until you find at least one that makes you fancy getting good at it. As you get better at whatever you have chosen, your increasing strength, skill, and endurance will begin to contribute to your self-concept in a way that equals the other things you do in your life that make you feel like a worthwhile person.

I hope you will take what I am saying very seriously because *our long-term follow-up of persons who have been in the Vanderbilt Weight Management Program shows that physical activity is likely to do more for your feeling of well-being and your physical self-concept than does weight loss*. Since this statement is particularly true for me, I'd like to tell you about the role that physical activity has played in my own successful fight against fat, and the continuing role that it plays in maintaining my health and good spirits. I know that it holds similar promise for you, if you will only give it a chance.

WHAT ACTIVITY HAS MEANT TO ME

I learned a great deal about what it takes to make physical activity an important part of one's daily life from personal experience. The very first thing I learned was its value in weight maintenance. I discovered that, after losing 15 or so pounds during my three weeks of dieting, I could return to my former food intake without gaining weight *provided* I played an hour and a half of singles tennis each day. I have measured my food intake over periods of several weeks, and it averages 2960 calories per day. I can say with a great deal of confidence that *nothing* works like physical activity for weight maintenance.

Without realizing it, however, I stumbled on to another very important key to the success of an activity program—the contribution it made to my self-concept.

All the while I was growing up as a fat child with about as poor a physical self-concept as anyone could have, I had an uncle who was an expert tennis player. He was my childhood idol. His name was Jules Daniels, and I watched him play with some of the best tennis players in the country. But Jules wouldn't even show me how to hold a racquet. I'm sure he felt that anyone as fat and klutzy as I was could never be a tennis player. And while I might have dreamed about becoming a tennis player, I never thought that it was possible, either.

My good old doctor friend, Ed Tarpley, changed all that when he said that I had to get active if I ever wanted to get my weight off, keep it off, and help prevent further heart problems. I remembered Uncle Jules and asked Ed if he would approve of tennis. He did, and he gave me the advice to start slowly and moderately.

I borrowed a tennis racquet and, together with the wife of one of my colleagues, went out in my street clothes to a tennis court near my office. I wanted to see if I had any talent for the game and if I could ever imagine myself getting good at it. I found, somewhat to my surprise, that I had much more coordination than I expected. Within a few days I was out on the court again, and within two weeks I was playing at least a half an hour every day. I began to have those dreams again of "being a tennis player" like my Uncle Jules.

I began to take tennis lessons and I was soon playing singles tennis every day for an hour and a half. Not only did it keep my weight down, but I began to look forward to those three weeks on my diet because each time I lost 15 pounds I could scamper around the court a great deal faster!

I played most of the time with players who were about equal to me in skill. That is the way to have the most fun and keep both participants interested. But I kept working at my game and improving. Finally, at the end of my first year, I got up the courage to ask one of Nashville's best players to hit with me. This man, Dr. Milt Bush, became one of my closest friends. In addition to being a well-known pharmacologist and a professor in the Pharmacology Department at Vanderbilt, Milt was, at that time, the part-time coach of the Vanderbilt tennis team. He was a nationally ranked player and his triumphs included both the United States Grass Courts Championship and the Canadian Open Clay Courts Championship when he was sixty-five years old.

One of the things that made Milt such an inspiration was that he won those national championships in spite of his having only one arm! If anyone knew what it means to conquer adversity, and to become a champion in spite of it, Milt did. I would meet him after team practice, and we would hit together. Occasionally he might drop a hint or two. My game began to improve by leaps and bounds.

• Soon I began to think of myself as "a tennis player." I wasn't playing for the sake of my health anymore, or for the weight-management benefits. These benefits became incidental to the effect tennis was having on the way I thought of myself as a person. There I was, "fat little Dicky," leaping around the court and winning tennis tournaments! The trophies became so numerous that I had to start storing them in the closet. People who have never been fat can never appreciate the thrill former fat persons experience when they discover their hidden physical talents and skills.

So this is what I mean about searching for a physical activity that can contribute to your self-concept. Perhaps you, too, have had a childhood dream about being an athletic person, but have felt too embarrassed to talk about it or pursue it.

Perhaps you, too, have had a secret idol who was a physically active person. I certainly hope that you, too, have dreamed of becoming a tennis player, or if not a tennis player, a dancer, a swimmer, or any other kind of active person. If you have had such dreams, or kindle them now, and if you then begin to engage in that activity, you will not have to worry about being fat EVER AGAIN. Being active will carry a value for you that is just as important to your sense of being worthwhile as the work you do for a living and the roles you play in your personal relationships as a father, mother, or servant to others in your community.

There is every likelihood that becoming active will lead you to find some new and special friends, just as I found Milt Bush.

For twenty years, up until his death a year ago at the age of seventy-seven, Milt and I looked forward to our weekly tennis match, and the couple of beers that followed, every Friday afternoon. It became a tradition, something so important and valuable in our lives that we felt deprived if anything interfered. Milt died in the way many tennis players would most prefer, of a heart attack in the middle of a tournament tennis match. I know that he preferred to exit his life in this way, because he had often told me of his desire never to linger here in poor health or to be limited in his physical and mental abilities. Today there is one trophy that doesn't get put away in my closet—it's the one Milt and I shared when we won the Music City Invitational Doubles Tournament here in Nashville several years ago. It stays on the mantel in the den and helps preserve the memory of a friendship I never would have known, and an experience I never would have had (winning that tournament with Milt), had I not made the attempt to become "a tennis player."

MAXIMIZING THE VALUE OF PHYSICAL ACTIVITY

When is the best time to be active?

How vigorous must I be?

Is it better to exercise for forty-five minutes all at once, or can I break it up?

How can I tell when any exercise—for example, swimming or bicycling—is equal to the weight-management benefits of forty-five minutes of brisk walking?

The Best Time to Exercise

The best time to exercise is when it feels the best to you, and is most convenient! Any other consideration is relatively minor. And as for the relative weight-management benefits of different activities, in general, brisk activity—of whatever kind—that involves moving your whole body through space, burns about 100 calories every fifteen minutes. Time of day can affect this value to the tune of about 5, or at the most, 10 percent.

However, since 5 or 10 percent of your daily expenditure in activity can equal enough calories to gain, or to *prevent* the gain of, a considerable amount of weight over time, you might want to consider the following guidelines.

You can get extra calorie-burning benefits if you exercise after eating. Your body has to work to digest your food. Normally, it takes about 10 percent of the caloric value of the food you eat to digest it. If you eat 1000 calories, the digestive process will take about 100 calories' worth of energy. However, you can increase by almost double the work it takes to digest food if you take a walk, *at a moderate pace,* after eating. Thus, if you need to walk back to work after a 1000-calorie lunch, and your walk is at least a mile in length, you will burn up about 200 calories in the digestive process. However, if you eat lunch near where you work, and there is no need to walk afterward, so that you just plop back in your chair after eating, you will use up only half that amount.

If you are one of those persons who has a great deal of difficulty losing weight, even on a very restricted diet, nothing will equal the value of adding some physical activity around mealtimes. Here is an example: if, before you ate, you had to walk fifteen minutes to reach the location where you were going to have lunch, and then, after eating, you had to walk fifteen minutes to return to work, the total *extra* energy that you would be expending would equal about 300 calories (200 involved in the walking itself, and another 100 over and above the usual cost of digestion). That is enough energy to keep about 40 to 50 pounds of fat *off* your body. Let me put it another way: if a person who normally did this amount of activity every day around mealtime were to stop, and did not change the level of food intake, he or she would gradually gain between 40 and 50 pounds during the next twelve to eighteen months!

As for time of day for physical activity—morning versus evening—the most convenient time is the best time, and the best time is whenever it feels best and suits you. Every other consideration is, once again, relatively minor.

At best, time of day can affect your caloric expenditure through exercise by an amount that's similar to the effect of walking after meals—about 5 to 10 percent. If you wish to obtain the benefit of burning an extra 5 to 10 calories for every brisk mile that you walk, exercising at the end of the day appears to be the way to do it. It works in the following way.

Late in the afternoon, your metabolic rate is likely to be at its highest point. This is a result of our inborn daily cycles of activity. If we wake and sleep according to the day-night cycle, our metabolic rate is lowest at about 5 A.M. and highest between 4 and 8 P.M. If we exercise when our metabolic rate is at a high point, the ceiling on energy expenditure seems to open up and we use more calories than usual. This, if you exercise before dinner, you may burn more calories than you might at five o'clock in the morning. I am happy to say that the effect seems to be greater for overweight persons than for normal-weight persons. Although time of day may amount to a small quantity on a daily basis, say 15 to 30 calories each day, on a year-round basis it can amount to several pounds.

If you happen to be a morning person, and by that I mean a person who wakes up and is, within moments, bursting with energy, I have a word of encouragement for morning exercise. In comparison with the evening person, your metabolic rate is already higher, and you can expect at least some extra calorie burning during your physical activity even in the morning.

Exercise Intensity

What do I mean by "brisk"?
Simply this:

First, be as vigorous as you can and not hurt yourself.

Second, be as vigorous as you can and still finish thirty to forty-five minutes of exercise feeling refreshed, not exhausted.

These are the principles that I use, and since I jog anywhere from 30 to 35 miles a week and have never had a running injury, I certainly feel confident in recommending them to all walkers and runners. In addition, since I almost always finish an hour's jog feeling more refreshed than when I started, I know that one doesn't have to work to exhaustion for weight control! So, just find your best cruising speed—one that you can maintain for whatever period you choose to be active.

(However, if you do decide to exercise intensely, that is, to the point where you are breathing very hard or actually get "out of breath" for a few moments at a time, be sure to "cool down" slowly. You should follow very intense activity with five minutes of moderate or gentle movement before stopping altogether. This cool-down will prevent the pooling of blood in your legs, reduce the burden on your heart, and help prevent cramping in your other working muscles.)

How Long Must You Exercise?

It is probably best to have one session each day of at least a half an hour in length. The reason I suggest that you try at least thirty minutes at a stretch is as follows.

If you move briskly and continuously for at least thirty minutes you may experience an elevation in your metabolic rate that can last several hours after you finish exercising. This "residual metabolic elevation" after a brisk walk can burn off between 50 and 100 calories more during the two to four hours after exercise than you would ordinarily burn following a period of inactivity. We have measured this effect in our laboratories, and in my own case, after an hour's jog, I tend to burn up over 10 percent more calories during the next six hours than I normally would burn if I had not been active.

There is another reason for exercising at least thirty minutes at a stretch—perhaps even forty-five or more—which is psychological in nature. It seems to take that long for your entire body to get into the rhythm of the movement. Walking, jogging, swimming, or bicycling in a safe place or indoors on a stationary bicycle begins to have meditational or hypnagogic effects after thirty or so minutes. When you enter into steady rhythmic movement, many physiological functions become coordinated in a steady state: breathing, heart rate, the movement of your arms and legs—in fact, the movement of almost all the major muscles of your entire body that are involved in maintaining your posture as you go through the various stages of each step. The refreshing, relaxing, "other-consciousness" effect is so great that yoga masters have, in fact, stated that meditation in motion (as in walking or jogging) is superior to meditation at rest. The so-called "runner's high," when it is experienced, seems to require at least forty-five minutes of continuous movement. Having tested many forms of meditation and many relaxation techniques, I can say that for me nothing can equal the refreshing, relaxing effects of an hour's gentle jog in the woods near my home.

But, once again, you have to decide what works best for you. As I indicated earlier, many persons who seem to be especially resistant to losing weight find that walking around mealtimes for fifteen-minute periods, three or four times each day, with two of these fifteen-minute walks right after meals, facilitates weight loss more than any other approach to activity.

If you have especially difficult problems in losing weight, you might try walking at mealtimes until you lose your weight. Then, get out there and work up to forty-five minutes of continuous activity of the kind I have just described. The ultimate psychological benefits of prolonged activity in one single period may then begin to outweigh all other considerations for you, as they do for me. And there is no question that single long periods of exercise work perfectly for long-term weight management.

Exercise and Appetite

Exercise has some additional beneficial weight-management effects on appetite. Although these benefits are valuable any time of the day, they seem especially useful for those many persons who pig out at night.

If you exercise at the end of the day, it may depress your nighttime eating urges. Exercise causes your liver to secrete glycogen and your fat cells to release fat. This increases the levels of sugar and fat in your bloodstream. Your brain senses this increase, which mimics the levels of fat and sugar in your bloodstream after eating, and it causes you to feel a decrease in appetite.

Exercise increases the level of epinephrine secretion from your adrenal glands. Epinephrine is a fat-mobilizing hormone: when you get active, epinephrine is released from your adrenal glands in order to stimulate your fat cells to release fat for energy. However, epinephrine is similar to amphetamine in its effects on appetite—it decreases your desire to eat. (One way you can recognize this effect is to notice the decrease in salivation that occurs during and after exercise.) Thus, when you exercise at the end of the day, you may experience a decrease in your appetite for the rest of the evening.

Finally, exercise at the end of the day may suppress night-time appetite in another way. Exercise elevates your body temperature. In fact, the internal body temperature of a person who has been engaging in vigorous physical activity can approach 104 degrees Fahrenheit. That's equivalent to a fever of considerable degree. Although you will feel great rather than ill after being active, this elevation in body temperature can have somewhat the same appetite-suppressing effects as the fever that accompanies illness.

I can vouch for the appetite-suppressing effects of evening exercise—and these effects are not always appreciated by my wife! She knows that it will be an hour or so before I feel like eating after a jog in the evening, and it sometimes annoys her to have to wait too long if we have planned to have dinner together. Keep this in mind if you begin to prefer evening exercise!

Although the appetite-suppressing effects of activity are great and worth working for, the emotional and psychological effects are even greater. I have already discussed some of these effects above. But there is even more for you to anticipate and experience. If you are now an inactive person, it may be hard for you to believe that, short of illness, *the more tired and aggravated you are before you get physically active, the better you will feel afterward*. Nothing will invigorate you and prepare you for a day of profitable work more than some brisk activity in the morning, and nothing will relax you and relieve you of the aggravations of a hard day at work more than some brisk activity before dinner. Indeed, it's at the end of the day, when you may feel drained of energy, that a brisk walk, jog, tennis match, or dance class is most elevating and refreshing, physically and mentally. Once you have experienced these effects, there is a good chance you will become addicted to your daily activity, and then it's really "bye-bye fat."

CAN YOU INCREASE YOUR METABOLIC RATE THROUGH EXERCISE?

Yes, you can. But you should be clear about what increasing your metabolic rate really means, both in principle and to you personally.

Simply put, your resting metabolic rate refers to the number of calories it takes to support a pound of your body weight for a given period of time, say, twenty-four hours (should you remain at rest for that period of time). Technically, metabolic rate is often calculated as calories burned per square meter of your body surface, but thinking in terms of a pound of body weight is easier to understand and more useful in weight management.

At the start of our program, we find that there is tremendous variability in the resting metabolic rates of our participants. A few persons, generally women, need fewer than 6 calories a day to maintain a pound of body weight in the resting state, whereas others, generally men, may need 9 or even 10 calories to maintain a pound of body weight in the resting state. Thus, a 200-pound person who needed, say, 7 calories per pound of body weight each day would have a resting need for 1400 calories, whereas another 200-pound person with a need for 10 calories per pound of body weight would need 2000 calories at rest over a twenty-four-hour period.

Men tend to have higher metabolic rates than women because, even when fat, they have as part of their total body weight a larger percentage of muscle tissue. Muscle tissue is considerably more active than fat tissue, even at rest—which means that muscle tissue burns more calories just maintaining itself—circulating nutrients and regenerating itself—then does fat tissue. Even at rest, muscle tissue may burn two or even three times more energy than does fat.

One way to change your resting metabolic rate is to change the composition of your body. That is, increase the amount of muscle tissue relative to the amount of fat. This will happen naturally by making sure that when you lose weight you lose only fat, or that, while losing weight, you slightly increase the amount of muscle on your body through appropriate exercise. In this way, when you calculate your metabolic rate, it will go up in terms of the calories you need each day per pound of weight.

I am happy to report that persons who get active in the manner I advise add, on the average, between 2 and 3 pounds of muscle for each 20 pounds lost. When you consider that up to half the weight you lose on diets without becoming active can be muscle tissue, this is an important advantage of the Rotation Diet and the activity program. If 10 of the 20 pounds lost on a diet are muscle tissue, you will be lowering, not increasing, your metabolic rate.

This becomes important when you consider the *total* number of calories it is going to take each day to maintain your weight at rest when you finish dieting. Here are the facts: *your total needs at rest are very likely to drop, in spite of an increase in the need per pound of weight!*

Think about it for a moment and you will see why: a given person who weighs 200 pounds at the start of a weight-loss campaign and loses 50 pounds, ending up with a body weight of 150 pounds, has a body to keep alive and move around each day that is 25 percent smaller. If that person needed 7 calories per pound of body weight before dieting, then the total daily need at rest would come to 1400 calories. If that person increased the need to 8 calories per pound of body weight at rest, which is, in fact, a considerable increase in metabolic rate, not likely to be obtained by many persons, the *total daily calorie need at rest would still end up at only 1200 calories.*

So you see, you can get an increase in metabolic *rate,* but, with a large amount of weight loss, an increase in rate is not likely to compensate completely for the loss in the *total* daily need for calories.

But think of the disaster that would occur for weight management if you not only lost weight, but also *lowered* your metabolic rate. If that 200-pound person whom I have been using as an example had even a slight decrease in metabolic rate (which would occur with the loss of muscle mass through dieting without becoming active)—say, down to 6½ calories per pound of body weight—at 150 pounds the total daily need would have fallen to 975 calories! Even if the needs had not changed, but remained the same at 7 calories per pound, the total need for calories would be reduced to 1050 at rest.

Now, of course, I think you see another reason why you must be active virtually every day for at least forty-five minutes to achieve permanent weight management. *It is during the forty-five minutes of brisk activity itself and during the residual metabolic elevation that can burn some additional calories when you finish being active that you burn up all the calories it used to take to keep alive all that extra fat you now have lost.*

And this is why I rant and rave—and why I will rant and rave once again, right here and now—against the dietmongers who want to sell you quick and easy weight-loss schemes without laying it all on the line and *demanding of you*, whenever physically possible, that you become an active person.

I cannot emphasize this too strongly: if you do not get active and stay active, you've got a snowball's chance in hell of maintaining any weight loss.

You will face semi-starvation for the rest of your life if you remain sedentary and want to control your weight. Just like everyone else in our affluent, overly nourished society, you are, and will be for life, surrounded by delicious, irresistable, high-calorie foods. Is it any wonder that 95 percent of dieters put their weight back on again?

I certainly hope you have an itchy feeling in your feet right now. So, go out for a walk, and then come back and read the next section on how to calculate the calories you burn in various physical activities.

HOW TO CALCULATE THE CALORIES BURNED IN PHYSICAL ACTIVITY

Compared with sitting at a desk, or lounging around watching TV, you will burn approximately three times more calories walking at a moderate pace (3 miles per hour).

When you work up to a brisk pace (4 miles per hour) you will burn almost five times more calories than you burn while sitting.

And if you lose enough weight to begin a little bit of gentle jogging, say, at a pace of a mile in ten minutes (6 miles per hour), you will burn between nine and ten times the calories you burn sitting still.

Table 7-1   Energy Expenditure in Physical Activities*

ACTIVITY	MINUTES OF ACTIVITY					
	5	10	15	30	45	60
Walking						
moderately, 3 miles per hour	22	44	66	132	198	264
briskly, 4 miles per hour	33	66	99	198	297	396
Rebounding**						
brisk walking tempo,						
little foot lift	22	44	66	132	198	264
jogging tempo,						
foot lift of 4–6 inches	33	66	99	198	297	396
running, high knee						
lifts, or kicks	68	136	204	408	612	816
Badminton	34	68	102	204	306	408
Cycling						
leisure, 5.5 miles per hour	22	44	66	132	198	264
leisure, 9.4 miles per hour	35	70	105	210	315	420
Chopping wood						
average tempo	30	60	90	180	270	360
Dancing						
moderate tempo	18	36	54	108	162	216
continuous, intense aerobic	59	118	177	354	531	708
Gymnastics	23	46	69	138	217	276
Horseback riding						
trot, English style	39	78	117	234	351	468
Martial arts, judo, karate						
continuous drill	68	136	204	408	612	816
Rowing						
moderate pace	26	52	78	156	234	312
Running (flat surface)						
a mile in 11½ minutes	47	94	141	282	423	564
a mile in 9 minutes	68	136	204	408	612	816
a mile in 8 minutes	73	146	219	436	655	874
a mile in 7 minutes	81	162	243	486	729	972
a mile in 6 minutes	88	176	264	528	792	1056
a mile in 5½ minutes	101	202	303	606	909	1212
Skiing						
moderate, downhill	42	84	126	252	378	504
cross country	50	100	150	300	450	600
Squash	74	148	222	444	666	888
Stair climbing						
down, rate of 1 step per second	17	34	51	102	153	204
up, rate of 1 step per second	72	144	216	432	648	864
Swimming						
continuous freestyle, slow	45	90	135	270	405	540
continuous freestyle, fast	55	110	165	330	495	660

ACTIVITY	MINUTES OF ACTIVITY					
	5	10	15	30	45	60
Table tennis	24	48	72	144	216	288
Tennis singles	38	76	114	228	342	456

*Estimates taken from Martin Katahn, *The 200 Calorie Solution,* Norton, 1982. All values are approximate for a person weighing 154 pounds.

**Rebounding exercise moves at a faster pace than walking on a level surface because of the assist given to your movement by the springing action of the minitrampoline.

Table 7-1 presents estimates of calories burned for the average 154-pound person in a number of different activities over different time periods. All estimates of this kind are rough, because of the great variability in our metabolic rates to begin with. The calories you end up burning in any activity are some multiple of this basal rate. A person who burns about 60 calories per hour at rest will burn approximately 300 calories per hour during a brisk walk. Another person, with a higher rate to begin with, say, 80 calories per hour, will end up burning around 400 per hour during a brisk walk.

Here is a rough rule of thumb that will do about as well as anything short of testing in a metabolic laboratory in predicting how many calories you burn in various activities.

If you do any whole-body activity that feels to you equivalent to walking at a moderate pace (3 miles per hour), you are likely to be burning somewhere between 225 and 325 calories an hour.

If you do any whole-body activity that feels to you equivalent to walking at a brisk pace (4 miles per hour), you are likely to be burning somewhere between 350 and 450 calories per hour.

If you do any whole-body movement that feels to you equivalent to gentle jogging (6 miles per hour), you will be burning somewhere between 650 and 750 calories per hour.

Women will burn fewer calories than men, and lighter persons fewer calories than heavier persons. A woman who weighs less than 120 pounds is quite likely to fall below the range I've suggested, whereas men over 200 pounds may exceed it.

I usually tell participants in my groups that there are two easy ways to think of the value of physical activity without getting obsessed with calories:

First, you will burn around 100 calories for every fifteen minutes of brisk activity. When you get into things that involve considerable running around, you will approach 150 calories burned every fifteen minutes.

Second, and the most important thing of all, is that in just forty-five minutes to one hour a day of physical activity you can burn 20 to 25 percent of your total daily intake of calories. This is a great way to have your cake and eat it, too, since it means you won't be adding an ounce of fat to your body and can eat like a normal human being without dieting.

THE VALUE OF PHYSICAL ACTIVITY IF YOU SUFFER FROM VARICOSE VEINS

I mentioned earlier in this book that I suffered from varicose veins even as a child and had my first attack of thrombophlebitis (blood clots and accompanying inflammation) at the age of twelve. Bouts with clots and inflammations continued to plague me throughout my life until about seven years ago. Losing weight and becoming a tennis player helped, but didn't completely prevent their occurrence.

But the attacks ceased entirely after I became a jogger.

The dramatic reduction in the problems I was having with my legs the moment I became a runner puzzled me, so I began to read about the effects of running on the circulation and the blood itself, and to ask questions of all my physician friends. This is what I discovered.

Continuous vigorous physical activity changes the clotting characteristics of the blood, increasing what is called fibrinolytic activity, which is one of the factors that reduces the tendency of the blood to clot. By jogging on an almost daily basis, I was remedying what has been a family tendency for generations. Tennis playing evidently either was not vigorous enough or did not involve enough sustained activity (as does jogging) to accomplish this result.

The effect of sustained physical activity on the characteristics of your blood is quite interesting. During intense activity, the ability of the blood to coagulate increases. This is a built-in tendency that serves to protect you, just in case you are injured. Evidently, when you stop and return to the resting state, there is a rebound in the other direction, so that at rest coagulation is less likely.

Of course you should not start to jog if you are overweight and suffer from varicose veins. But I suggest you discuss the following total program for self-care with your physician. From what I have learned in my study of the problem, I believe that about 50 percent of persons who suffer from varicose veins, phlebitis, and thrombophlebitis will benefit tremendously from following it. Your varicose veins will not go away, but they are not nearly as likely to hurt or become inflamed, nor is your blood as likely to clot, if you put this program into effect.

A PREVENTION PROGRAM FOR OVERWEIGHT PERSONS WHO SUFFER FROM VARICOSE VEINS

Except where noted, there is scientific evidence to support the help you can receive by following each of these preventive steps. The first and the last steps are probably the most important beneficial changes that you can make in caring for yourself.

1. Get down to ideal weight.

2. Do not eat large meals (it can interfere with circulation to your legs).

3. Do not wear obstructive, tight-fitting clothing for the same reason.

4. Do not eat high-fat meals, which clog your blood with a high fat content. (I do not have strong evidence that high-fat meals will slow the blood flow and increase clotting in your veins, although there is very strong evidence that a high-fat diet, especially a diet high in the saturated fat that comes from meat products, is correlated with deposits of fatty substances on the walls of the coronary arteries and with coronary heart disease. This is purely intuitive advice on my part.)

5. Do not stand in one place for more than a few minutes at a time—keep moving. Flexing your calf muscles aids circulation. Flexing also helps when you have to sit in one place for a long period.

6. Elevate your legs at every opportunity to assist the flow of blood back to your heart.

7. Raise the leg end of the mattress you sleep on so it is about two inches higher than your waist (you can fold a blanket and slip it under the mattress).

8. If you should suffer from gnawing pains in your legs at night, turn around in bed, put your legs up over the headboard, and stay that way for about fifteen minutes to let blood drain from your legs. You can also do a backstand: rest on your back on the floor or bed, lift your legs and hips to the vertical position, supporting yourself with your hands on your hips, and hold this position for several minutes. Your weight will rest on the backs of your upper arms from the elbows to the shoulders. However, if you have high blood pressure, check with your doctor about the advisability of these positions before you attempt to do either of them.

9. At the first sign of any problem, elevate your legs and gently massage them, with the motion going toward your heart. If you do not have an anti-inflammatory drug at hand, take one aspirin tablet and get in touch with your physician.

10. If you receive any sort of bruise to your legs that might cause an inflammation or a clot, put an ice pack on it immediately.

11. Be careful in the use of elastic stockings or bandages. Sometimes these can obstruct circulation and hurt, rather than help, the condition. If you need to use support hose, experiment until you find the very best possible style for your condition. You need to talk this over with your doctor, and be sure to tell him what effects the support you are presently using are having. If there is pain, the support hose are probably not helping, and may be doing additional damage. No matter who prescribed or fitted them, when support hose begin to hurt, get them off immediately and get in touch again with your physician. You may need another prescription.

12. *Above all, as you lose your weight, begin to gradually increase your walking.* I believe that vigorous walking *worked up to in both speed and time very gradually to the forty-five minutes per day that I am recommending,* will accomplish the same thing for you

that jogging has done for me. However, as long as you are overweight, you must be very moderate and very careful, or you can aggravate, rather than help, the condition.

To gain the most benefit from continuous vigorous physical activity, and to be able to pursue it with more benefits than risk for varicose veins, you must be at the very best weight that you can possibly achieve.

All of my suggestions are designed to prevent or to minimize trouble with varicose veins. My suggestions are not a *treatment* for phlebitis, thrombophlebitis, and varicose veins. These are medical conditions that require medical treatment. While I have not needed them in years, I still carry with me, in my tennis bag and in my suitcase on trips, the blood thinner, the clot-dissolving enzyme, and the anti-inflammatory drug that my physician has prescribed in case of trouble. You need medical supervision, too, but discuss the preventive measures I have just described with your doctor. I believe that they can help you, as they have helped me, prevent inflammations and clots and that they will lessen a very aggravating problem.

8

Taking a Vacation from Dieting: The Transition To Maintenance

Why do you have to stop now and take a vacation from dieting? If you have more weight to lose, why can't you just continue using the Rotation Diet over and over again until you lose all the weight you need to lose?

And, if you have reached your goal weight, why do you have to make a "transition" to maintenance? If you haven't lowered your metabolic rate and reduced your need for food, why can't you begin your celebration immediately and eat anything and everything you want to eat right away, without gaining weight?

The answers to the questions in the first paragraph are quite simple and brief: there are four reasons why you have to take a vacation from dieting, and they are all equally important.

First, a break in dieting guarantees that there will be no slowdown in metabolic rate.

Second, the break increases your motivation to be as perfect as possible during each three-week period that you use the Rotation Diet. Longer periods of dieting encourage small deviations, followed by larger deviations, finished off by complete collapse.

Third, if you have problems controlling your appetite, you

are not as likely to begin to overeat after only three weeks of dieting (especially because of that little respite during the second week) as you are if you had forced yourself to endure several more weeks or months of deprivation. Long periods of dieting build up powerful hidden impulses to binge.

Fourth, you need the practice maintaining small weight losses on your way to complete success. It is much easier to manage maintenance after three separate 10- or 15-pound losses than it is to manage your weight after losing 30 to 45 pounds all at once. With each 10- or 15-pound loss you discover what you need to do with your diet and activity program, and you begin to incorporate the metabolic benefits that go with increased physical activity and improvements in your diet. You already have learned some of the things you need to do to raise your metabolic rate and to increase your total daily metabolic needs in previous chapters. I will discuss some additional metabolic benefits that you can obtain from improving the quality of your diet later in this chapter.

Now to answer the questions in the second paragraph. Why do you have to make a "transition" to maintenance? Why can't you eat anything you want right now, immediately after finishing the Rotation Diet?

The reason is water retention.

Because we tend to blame "water retention" for a number of things when our weight fluctuates, I think you should be clear about the way your body varies in its water balance, apparently whimsically (but really lawfully) increasing and decreasing its total water content, while still tending to hover around some central point. There are a number of factors involved in causing these fluctuations, and they can all come into play and affect your weight at any time, including this period when you must take a vacation from dieting.

First of all, haven't you noticed how your body weight tends to jump around within a range of about 3 to 5 pounds over a one- to three-day period? For example, take a time when you are not on a reducing diet. You go out to a party on a Sunday evening, have a couple of glasses of wine, some snack food, perhaps a rich main course, and then dessert. You wake up 3 pounds heavier the next morning. In order to gain a true 3 pounds of *fat* weight, you would have had to eat about 10,500 calories *more* than your normal intake. (Each pound of body fat contains about 3500 calories.) You know darn well you haven't binged to that extent. You may have had 1500 extra calories, but certainly not 10,500. How can you gain 3 pounds on 1500 calories?

Now take the opposite situation. It's the middle of the week, you haven't been on a reducing diet, you haven't been around any desserts or alcohol, and you have been too busy to cook anything except plain food. Perhaps, in addition, you ran out of salty snack foods. Over a three-day period you may have eaten 500 calories a day less than you did over the last weekend. Now, on Thursday morning, you find yourself 3 pounds lighter than you were on Monday. What accounts for this?

As I indicated, it's a question of water balance.

The human body is, on the average, about 72 percent water. This means that a person weighing about 140 pounds has a body that contains about 100 pounds of water. Muscle tissue, for example, is 75 to 80 percent water, blood is almost 100 percent water, and the sugar energy stores in your liver (glycogen) are dissolved in a ratio of one part sugar to three or four parts water. In addition, there is a considerable amount of fluid all around our body cells. Thus, given 100 pounds or more of water in our bodies, it is easy to imagine that there are many different factors that might cause the body to vary by 3 to 5 percent (3 to 5 pounds) in its water content, overnight.

SOME FACTORS AFFECTING WATER BALANCE

Sodium

Most of us know, of course, about the effects of the sodium in table salt and in monosodium glutamate (MSG). Sodium is one of the nutrients that can cause a major amount of water retention when we take in more than our kidneys can dispose of quickly. There is enough sodium in just one medium-sized pickle to cause a 1-pound weight gain in susceptible persons. And, since most persons who have a weight problem also tend to retain more than the average amount of water, I tell participants in our program that it's "a pound a pickle." Similarly, if you have what is essentially a low-calorie Chinese meal, you can show a 2- or 3-pound weight gain the next morning without having overeaten by one single calorie. The gain is due primarily to the sodium in the MSG and, possibly, to the overuse of soy sauce.

Changes in Calorie Intake

Although you may be aware of the effects of too much sodium on your body-weight, you may not understand how an increase in the caloric content of a day's food intake *of only 500 calories* more than was eaten the previous day can also lead to a 1-pound weight gain. The body responds to a change in caloric intake just as it would to a dose of sodium, and, up to a total of about 2000 calories more than your usual intake, you can gain weight at about 1 pound for each 500 extra calories.

Most people give themselves the double whammy when they go off the deep end and begin to overeat. They combine an increase in sodium consumption (high in most dip and snack foods) with an increase in calories. Overeat by 500 calories each day for three days (or stuff in 1500 extra calories in one day) and, in addition, fail to watch your sodium intake, and you can easily gain 5 pounds. This sort of weight gain is especially likely to happen to sedentary persons because they do not do anything in the way of physical activity that can get rid of some water via perspiration and respiratory activity.

You can see the most dramatic illustration of rebound water retention (technically called "the rehydration effect") after a diet in persons who have stopped all food intake and who have been on a complete fast in order to lose weight. A few years ago I visited one of our country's famous fasting programs and watched obese men who had just finished three weeks of fasting in a medically supervised program gain 7 pounds in five days on a refeeding diet *of only 600 calories per day!* Since the average loss was under 20 pounds this meant they were regaining weight faster than they had lost it.

Stress, Overexertion, and Alcohol

Two other factors that can cause several pounds of water retention, without overeating, are severe stress, which I hope you will never face at any time of your life, and physical activity at a high intensity or prolonged duration, to which you are not accustomed.

With respect to stress, weight gains of 6 or 7 pounds have been noted in persons experiencing the onset of divorce proceedings, the death of a person dear to them, or a war. And after unusually hard exercise, you may overshoot the mark in your fluid intake. In addition, any inflammation of your muscles and joints following unusually intense or prolonged exercise will be associated with fluid retention.

Temporary water retention is a very common occurrence among active persons who suddenly increase their level of activity. It has happened to me. The very first time that I ran an eight-mile course, which was three miles farther than I had ever run before, I expected to be lighter the next day. In spite of not having overeaten, I gained 2 pounds instead. It took me a while to associate the gain with the amount of fluid I had drunk, and the slight soreness in my leg muscles and joints. Of course, temporary water-weight gains as a result of overexercising are not seen in persons who maintain a rather steady exercise program. Normally, exercise is an important element in eliminating excess water retention.

Finally, the use of alcohol leads to water retention in many people. Even beer drinkers! You may spend the whole night running to the bathroom as you drink your beer, but you are likely to end up retaining more water than you started with.

Although the Rotation Diet has given you a quick weight loss without predisposing you to a rebound gain in your *fat* weight, you are still just as susceptible as you ever were to a temporary but terribly discouraging gain due to water retention, *unless* you follow my guidelines for making a transition to maintenance. And, by the way, these guidelines are generally effective in preventing water retention due to any cause, including periodic water retention during the menstrual cycle, and they will help keep you from bloating whether or not you are on a diet. In any event, I know just how discouraging an overnight gain of several pounds can be, so let's be sure it doesn't happen to you!

GUIDELINES FOR MAKING
A SUCCESSFUL TRANSITION
TO MAINTENANCE

The first thing I want to say is, DON'T WORRY. You will be able to eat again like a normal human being and not gain weight! You will be able to return to the style of cooking you prefer (unless it was loaded with fat!), you will be able to eat out and, while eating out, be able to eat as others eat. But you must follow each of my guidelines. You cannot go off the deep end and immediately binge to celebrate all the weight you have lost. And you can *never* return to a sedentary life-style (assuming you have increased your activity level) without endangering your weight. You have just got to keep burning up, on a daily basis, all the calories it used to take to keep the fat you have just lost alive on your body, or it will start creeping back!

Increase Food Intake Slowly

Of all the guidelines, this is probably the most important. If you increase food intake too quickly, you will probably increase both calories *and* sodium. Assuming that you have just completed the twenty-one days of the Rotation Diet, do not increase your food intake to more than 1200 calories for each of the next three days if you are a woman, and 1800 calories a day if you are a man.

To make the transition to maintenance as easy as possible, we suggest that women in the Vanderbilt Weight Management Program use the 1200-calorie menus of Week 2 of the Rotation Diet (page 52), and men the 1800-calorie menus (page 58).

If you want to be absolutely sure you will not gain weight, use the Week 2 menus for a whole week. When our participants use the Week 2 menus for a full week, they usually lose about two more pounds. You may do this too, if you like, since it gives some insurance against water retention when you add more calories next week. The two additional pounds that you lose in the fourth week after beginning the Rotation Diet will be ALL fat loss.

After women have been on the 1200-calorie menus for at

least three days (or a week, if you prefer), they should increase to 1500 calories. Stick with 1500 calories for three days, using the 1500-calorie menus that I have laid out for men (pages 58–61, and pages 191–194 in the Alternate Menus), if you wish to make it easy for yourself.

With daily brisk activity of at least forty-five minutes, women should be able to reach a daily intake of around 1800 calories sometime during the fifth week after beginning the Rotation Diet. Use my 1800-calorie menus as guides (pages 58–61, and pages 194–199 in the Alternate Menus). You can, if you like, consider this week your "vacation from dieting" and start all over again next week. But I always took at least a month off between rotations and you may be happier and more successful if you do the same. It gives you practice in maintenance and keeps motivation at peak levels.

After spending three to seven days on 1800 calories, men also go up by 300-calorie increments, first to 2100 calories for three days, then to 2400 calories.

Thus, no matter what your sex, you see that you must think in terms of 300-calorie increments until you determine where your weight will stabilize with your new level of physical activity. Since we are all different, it must necessarily be a testing process.

For those of you who don't wish to follow my menus, and for men going up to 2100 and 2400 calories, to be on the safe side I would suggest adding only extra servings of fruits, vegetables, and lean meat, fowl, or fish to meet the 300-calorie increases. You can build your own menus using my recipes, since these recipes will give you the calorie contents for each serving. For other foods, see the calorie guide on pages 227–233 for quick calorie estimates. In general, note the following:

Half-cup servings of all vegetables except *free vegetables* will contain around 25 calories.

The average-size piece of fruit will run around 60 calories, with small fruits (such as a plum) containing around 40 calories and large fruits (a large apple) containing about 80 calories.

You can consider *lean* meats, fish, and fowl to contain about 55 calories per ounce, and you will not be far from correct. But watch out for the fat! Fatty meats can run over 100 calories per ounce.

What about the "goodies": desserts, candy, alcohol?

If you choose to include dessert, snack foods, or alcohol, rather than the fruits, vegetables, and lean meat, fish, or fowl that are preferable when you first increase calories, you should add only one serving of such foods on any given day, until you determine just how such increases affect your weight. Since no one can predict exactly what will happen until it's tried, it's up to you to find out for yourself. If your weight goes up on just one serving, you can be absolutely certain that it is due to water retention. It is impossible to gain a pound of fat on one serving of any dessert or one glass of wine! (You may gain more than a pound of water if you get into salty snacks, however. But again, it is not a gain in fat weight.)

If you use all of the other guidelines that I give you in this chapter, you should not gain a single pound during your transition to maintenance. If you gain any weight at all, you will stabilize at a point very close to your lowest weight. Then, if you eliminate, *for just one day,* all of the dessert foods, alcohol, and salty snacks that put you at the high point in your water balance, that increase in water weight will drop off just as quickly as it was gained. Working in this way you can find out how susceptible you are to water retention from desserts, alcoholic beverages, and salt, and you can be certain that as you add or eliminate them from your diet you are simply playing with a pound or two of water weight.

Are there some foods that affect your metabolic rate, so that eating them can elevate that rate and help you stay thin?

Yes, there is a way that the food you eat affects your total metabolic needs and it is *very important* for you to understand how it works so you can put the principles to work in order to help you maintain your losses in the future. But that is a long-term rather than a short-term matter, and it needs some detailed explanation, so I will wait until the end of this chapter to discuss it. Right now I want to give you the other guidelines for making the transition to maintenance without gaining any weight—even water weight.

Avoid Excess Salt

A bowl of onion soup, a couple of tablespoons of blue cheese dressing, a couple of pickles to go with a salami sandwich, and you will be a few pounds heavier tomorrow morning.

Don't cook with salt—add it to taste at the table. And learn to use herbs and spices as I suggest in my many recipes.

Here is a list of foods high in sodium. Eliminate those that have no nutritional value and eat those that do in moderation. For example, be moderate in your consumption of most cheeses. They are an important source of calcium, but they also tend to be high in sodium (see page 65 for a comparison of the sodium content of some popular cheeses). Avoid foods that contain not much more than just sodium and fat (for example, bacon and sausage) and prepare the foods that appear in this list which are normally nutritious foods, without the salt that has been used in the noted method of preparation (for example, beef and fish are normally nutritious foods, but corned beef and smoked fish are prepared with excess salt).

anchovies and anchovy paste
bacon
baking powder
baked beans with pork
beef, corned, dried
bouillon cubes (except low sodium; check label)
canned vegetables
catsup in large quantities
celery salt (celery *seed* is fine)
cereals (check label; the best ones will have less than 250 milligrams per serving)
cheese (blue, cheddar, processed)
codfish, smoked and salted
corn, popped with salt added (okay plain)
crab, canned

crackers, soda type
ham
olives
peanuts, salted
pickles
potato chips and other similarly salted snack foods
processed luncheon meats
pretzels, salted
sauerkraut
sausage, frankfurters
soups, canned
soy sauce (1 teaspoon of soy sauce has about 285 milligrams of sodium; 1 teaspoon of salt has 2000 milligrams of sodium)
TV dinners (check labels)
Worcestershire sauce

Eat Naturally Diuretic Foods

Some foods have a natural diuretic function. They stimulate your kidneys to rid your body of water, rather than close them down as do the salty foods just listed. Naturally diuretic foods tend to be relatively high in potassium content, compared with their sodium content.

Here is a list of foods that will help you get rid of excess water. The most effective ones seem to be fresh pineapple, asparagus, citrus fruits, and green vegetables. Combine these foods with lean meat and cottage cheese, and you can lose several pounds of water overnight.

apricot	milk, skim and low-fat
asparagus	nuts, unsalted
banana	pineapple, fresh
beef, lean	potato
broccoli	prunes and prune juice
cantaloupe	oranges and orange juice
chicken	raisins
cottage cheese	tomato
figs	tuna, water packed
grapefruit and grapefruit juice	turkey
lamb, trimmed	watermelon

ONE-DAY WATER-LOSS DIET

Just in case you ever experience water retention, here is a day's menu that will get rid of several pounds of excess water. Women who experience periodic water retention find it particularly helpful, especially when it is combined with the daily exercise that I recommend. It will also do wonders for your mood since water retention is often associated with an increase in negative emotions such as depression.

Up to 1 pound of extra-lean beef, fish, or chicken, prepared without skin

Up to 2 cups of low-fat cottage cheese

Asparagus, broccoli, fresh pineapple or melon, and citrus fruits

You can use this diet for two days if necessary, and you can eat up to a full pound of lean meat, fish, or fowl and 2 cups of low-fat cottage cheese each day. You can also eat all the named fruits and vegetables, plainly cooked, in almost unlimited quantities. To be on the safe side, however, the first time you use the diet, try a serving each of two different vegetables, and a serving each of two different fruits. This will show you how well the diet can work for you when followed in its most perfect form.

If you have been retaining an extreme amount of water, you can lose 5 or more pounds on the One-Day Water-Loss Diet. Although I do not normally retain fluid, I have tried this diet after a big weekend and lost 3¾ pounds. The combination of a high protein content together with naturally diuretic fruits and vegetables does it. But do not use a diet such as this for more than two days. Over longer periods of time, you should eat a wide variety of foods to assure yourself of adequate nutrition.

Be Physically Active

DON'T MISS A DAY! If you are in good health, by the time you make this transition to maintenance you will be walking briskly for forty-five minutes a day, or engaging in some other physical activity. Between the activity itself and the residual elevation in your metabolic rate that stays with you for a few hours after your activity, you will be burning off between 300 and 400 more calories each day than you did before you began the Rotation Diet. As you begin to increase your calories to stabilize your weight, your new activity level will be burning off enough calories to keep the fat you lost during the three weeks of the Rotation Diet from ever returning to your body.

Almost as important as the fat-burning power of physical activity is its aid in preventing water retention. Normally, on any given day, we lose almost as much water through perspiration and respiration as we do through the kidneys. (Our breath is 100 percent saturated with moisture when we exhale.) When we are active, we can lose one to several pounds of water through perspiration, and, as we increase our breathing rate, we can double the loss of moisture through respiration. *You can retain several pounds of water on any day that you skip your activity session*. So, it is absolutely essential that you maintain your activity level during the transition to weight maintenance.

Drink Eight Glasses of Water Daily

I repeat these directions because drinking eight 8-ounce glasses of water daily is as important to weight maintenance as it is to weight loss. *Don't make the mistake of thinking that cutting back on water can prevent water retention*. Just the opposite! Adequate fluid intake stimulates the kidneys and helps to reduce water retention, and your body has to burn some calories in the process. In addition, adequate water intake will keep you regular and prevent the gain of a pound or two of refuse weight. Always use water in place of the dietetic beverages you might have used in the past. This will help prevent the reawakening of your sweet tooth!

Remember Your Safe Fruit

Perhaps the one most important dietary change that has stayed with me in my twenty-two years of weight maintenance has been the substitution of fruit as snacks and desserts for junk foods and other dense-calorie foods (foods high in fat and sugar). I have mentioned previously how I nibble on fruit all day long—it's many different kinds now, not just grapefruit, and it's really not quite all day long, just two or three snacks. Right now, in a large bowl, right out in plain sight in the kitchen, is a very attractive selection of grapes (two kinds), oranges, the crisp York apples that have just come into season, bananas, and grapefruit. I can eat to my heart's content, never be hungry, and never worry about being fat again.

I think you, too, will find weight maintenance a snap if you substitute "safe fruit" (that is, all fresh fruit) for your previous snack foods. Similarly, if you make a practice of eating all kinds of fruits, including dried fruits of all kinds, for desserts, in place of pies, cakes, and cookies, you will have your weight problem licked. Try it. Make a fruit substitution for processed snack foods and for most of your desserts (not all, of course—you will find that that isn't necessary in maintenance). I guarantee that you will feel a great deal better as well as be a success in maintenance when you substitute fruit for most of the "junk food" that might now be in your diet. Fruit substitutions are great for your digestive processes and will go a long way to help you deal with your sweet tooth, if you have one. (For a deeper understanding of the "junk-food" problem, and a definition of "junk food," see the additional discussion on pages 167–169.)

There you have it. I know that you have worked hard to lose the weight you have lost. Having been on the yo-yo myself during the first thirty-five years of my life, before I found out how to maintain my own weight loss, I know how frustrating it can be to let your weight start creeping up again. Follow my guidelines in making your transition to maintenance and you, too, will achieve permanent weight control. Here they are, once again, in summary form:

---

1. Increase Food Intake Slowly
2. Avoid Salt and Salty Foods
3. Eat Naturally Diuretic Fruits and Vegetables
4. Be Physically Active on a Daily Basis
5. Drink Eight 8-ounce Glasses of Water a Day
6. Make All Fruit Your "Safe Fruit" and Substitute Them for the Junk Food in Your Diet

---

Now we are ready to discuss the *permanent* metabolic benefits that you can obtain by making one very significant change in the quality of your diet.

HOW TO INCREASE YOUR METABOLIC NEEDS WITH DIET

Although a calorie is a calorie in the laboratory, all calories are not the same to the human body.

For a long time even the best, most informed nutritionists claimed that it didn't matter where your calories came from. They said that all calories meant the same thing in terms of energy to the human body. Recent research disproves this statement.

Fat, for example, is easily converted to a form that your body can use for energy, and it's very easy to convert dietary fat to *body* fat for storage. It is especially easy to gain weight if you happen to eat more fat than your daily energy requirements.

Carbohydrates and protein need a great deal more digestive work to convert their energy than does fat, and this results in a "wasting" of some of the energy. That is, while the calorie count for a carbohydrate or protein food may be accurate in your calorie book, your body doesn't end up using all the listed calories for energy in vital processes. Some of the calories are burned up and thrown off as heat.

Similarly, if you should overeat on either carbohydrates or protein, the body has to work much harder to change these nutrients into fat than it does to change dietary fat into body fat.

In fact, it takes between four and five times more energy to convert carbohydrate and protein to fat than to convert dietary fat to body fat.

Perhaps this will become intuitively evident if you just imagine a quantity equal to two teaspoons of fat or oil sitting in a dish next to a fairly large apple. Both food items will be about equal in calories as measured in the laboratory apparatus that determines how many calories they each contain (about 70 to 80 calories). But your body will have to work a lot harder to change the calories in that apple into body fat than it has to work to change the calories in that fat or oil into body fat.

It takes about 5 percent of the energy content of dietary fat to convert it to body fat. It takes 20 to 25 percent of the energy in carbohydrate and protein to turn these nutrients into body fat.

Obviously, if you substitute carbohydrate or protein calories for fat calories, you can end up eating many calories more and still not gain any weight. Even though your total calorie count is up, you have increased your metabolic needs by making the body work harder in the process of digestion. So, you don't gain any weight.

Other Values of a Diet Low in Fat and High in Dietary Fiber

There are two other factors that prevent weight gain when you increase complex carbohydrates in your diet (whole grains, fruits, and vegetables) and decrease fats.

First, these foods, and only these foods, contain dietary fiber. Fiber is included in the calorie counts in your calorie books, but the body doesn't digest these calories! Our stomachs and intestines don't have the appropriate enzymes to break down that fiber (other animals do). So, depending on the particular carbohydrate foods you eat, perhaps 10 percent or even more of the total listed calories passes right through your system as roughage.

Second, as an extra metabolic benefit, the fiber contained in the complex carbohydrates will tangle up about 10 percent of the dietary fat you eat, and that, too, will pass right through your system without being digested.

So, can you, in fact, "increase your metabolism through eating?" If you substitute complex carbohydrates for fats in your diet, the answer is yes. If you cut your fat consumption in half, and, instead, start eating fresh fruits and vegetables and whole-grain products, you will end up needing a couple of hundred extra calories each day, over and above what you are presently eating, just to maintain your present body weight. This amounts to a considerable increase in your total daily metabolic needs.

YOU HAVE NOW DISCOVERED THE MAGICAL CURE FOR OBESITY

I have taken a great many pages to explain the details of the Rotation Diet and to show you how you can make a transition to maintenance that will keep off all the weight you have lost in the last three weeks. If you have more weight to lose, after a week's or a month's vacation from dieting (it's up to you), go back on the diet.

When you reach your desired weight, you also know a magical cure for obesity that will prevent every single pound of lost fat from ever reaccumulating on your body. The magical cure for obesity—everything I have said in this book, in fact, that leads to permanent weight management—can be boiled down to five little words:

EAT LESS FAT AND WALK

In the next three chapters I will tell you some things you can do from both a practical and a psychological standpoint to put this magical cure to work on a permanent basis. I wish there were some way around it, but the magical cure is not a one-time remedy—it only works when you use it on a daily basis.

9

The Weight-Mastery Quiz: Testing Your Weight-Management Confidence

At the first meeting with new participants in the Vanderbilt Weight Management Program I do something that may seem a little strange: I give each person a delicious bar of milk chocolate for their very own! This is not meant to be some kind of sadistic joke. It is, in fact, the first step toward complete mastery over their appetite for foods that have stimulated them to overeat.

I am going to show you how to achieve the same mastery for yourself, which you can do on your own by following the same procedures that we use in our program. Before I do this, here is a quiz that will identify your most serious weight-management problems and the areas of weight management in which you have the least confidence in your ability to succeed.

WEIGHT-MASTERY QUIZ*

Directions: Here are descriptions of three typical situations in each of six areas that present major weight-management problems for overweight persons. Imagine yourself in each situation (or think of one from your own experience that is similar to it, which you are likely to encounter on a frequent basis). Then, rate the confidence you have in your ability to carry out the behavior that would lead to greater control over your weight problem. Use a scale that ranges from 0 to 100 percent confidence. If you have a complete lack of confidence in yourself—that is, you feel that you would never be able to act appropriately—give yourself a 0. If you think that you might respond correctly about 50 percent of the time, give yourself a 50. And, if you feel that you have complete confidence, give yourself a rating of 100 percent. For convenience in scoring, do not use intervals smaller than 5 percent (50, 55, 60, etc.) in making your ratings.

Problem Area Number 1: Resisting Temptation

CONFIDENCE RATING

1. It's 5:30 P.M. and you are in the middle of preparing a delicious dinner. How confident are you that you will wait until the meal is served before eating anything?

_____

2. You are spending an evening home alone and you are tempted to snack on a high-calorie food. How confident are you that you will resist the urge to snack?

_____

3. You are watching TV and some high-calorie snack foods (cookies, chips, soft drinks, beer, etc.) are brought into the room. How confident are you that you will watch TV without eating a high-calorie snack?

_____

---

*This quiz is based on a questionnaire developed by Dr. David Schlundt, Department of Psychology, Vanderbilt University, Nashville, TN 37240, and adapted with his collaboration for research in the Vanderbilt Weight Management Program. You may obtain the complete research version by writing directly to Dr. Schlundt and asking for the diet questionnaire. Please enclose $1.00 to cover the postage and handling expenses.

Problem Area Number 2: Social Eating

4. You are having dinner with your family   CONFIDENCE
and someone picks up the platter that contains a   RATING
favorite dish, and says, "Let me give you a little
more," and begins to fill your plate. How confident are you that you will be able to say "No,
thanks" and stick with your food plan?   _____

5. You are at a party for a friend and someone offers you a slice of cake, or other high-calorie
food that is not on your food plan. How confident
are you that you will turn it down?   _____

6. You enjoy a good celebration and are out
to dinner at a fine restaurant with friends. How
confident are you that you will celebrate without
overeating?   _____

Problem Area Number 3: Food Choice

7. You have finished dinner and the choice of
fruit or cake (or some other high-calorie dessert) is
available. How confident are you that you will
choose fruit instead of cake?   _____

8. You prefer to prepare high-calorie meals
(flavoring with butter or other fat, frying foods,
using sauces that are high in calories). How confident are you that you will prepare low-calorie
dishes instead?   _____

9. You are out to eat in a fine restaurant that
offers you a choice of both low-calorie and high-
calorie dishes at every course. How confident are
you that you will make *only* low-calorie choices?   _____

Problem Area Number 4. Exercise

10. You have begun an exercise program, but
find that family, friends, or business obligations

begin to make demands and interfere. How confident are you that you will stick with your daily exercise program?

_____

11. You are asked by another person to go for a walk (or engage in some other physical activity), but you are feeling tired and kind of low. How confident are you that you will overcome these feelings and say yes to the walk (or other activity)?

_____

12. You plan to exercise after work today (or at the end of the day, before dinner) but you feel tired and hungry when the time arrives. How confident are you that you will exercise anyway?

_____

Problem Area Number 5: Overeating

13. You are at a party surrounded by tasty, high-calorie foods. You have already eaten more than you should, but are tempted to continue. How confident are you that you will stop eating right now?

_____

14. Instead of putting food away after a meal, you find yourself eating the leftovers. How confident are you that you will put the food away without eating any?

_____

15. You overeat at supper when you are tired and hungry when you get home. How confident are you that you will not overeat?

_____

Problem Area Number 6: Negative Emotions

16. You crave things to eat when you are lonely, blue, or bored. How confident are you that you will find another way to cope with these feelings and not overeat?

_____

17. You have just had an argument with a family member and you are upset and angry. You are standing in front of the refrigerator and you feel like eating everything in sight. How confident are you that you will find some other way to make yourself feel better?

_____

18. You are anxious and tense after a very trying day. You have the urge to get a candy bar (piece of pie, cake, etc.). How confident are you that you will find a more constructive way to calm down and cope with your feelings?

CONFIDENCE RATING

_____

Scoring

Score yourself in the following way. How many of the three items within each of the six problem categories receive confidence ratings of 50 percent or less, 55 to 70 percent, 75 to 85 percent, or 90 percent or greater? Write down the number in the chart below.

CATEGORY	NUMBER OF ITEMS RECEIVING:			
	50 percent or less	55 to 70 percent	75 to 85 percent	90 percent or greater
Resisting Temptation	_____	_____	_____	_____
Social Eating	_____	_____	_____	_____
Food Choice	_____	_____	_____	_____
Exercise	_____	_____	_____	_____
Overeating	_____	_____	_____	_____
Negative Emotions	_____	_____	_____	_____

Interpreting Category Scores

If your ratings of any two of the three questions in a category fall within the two lowest levels of confidence, either the 50 percent or less level or the 55 to 70 percent level, this is a problem area that is likely to pose an extreme threat to your weight-management efforts.

Any category in which two of the three ratings fall _below_ the highest level of confidence (90 percent or greater) is likely to pose a less serious, but still significant, problem area.

Any category that receives two or more ratings in the 90 percent or greater level of confidence is not, as a problem area considered in its entirety, likely to pose a major threat to weight management. However, a low confidence rating in any specific situation must be dealt with if that situation occurs with great frequency.

Interpreting Individual Items

Low ratings on individual questions can be very significant, even though your confidence in the two related situations within the same category of weight-management problems is higher. This is particularly true, as I have just indicated, if you must face that situation frequently. Anything less than a 90 percent confidence rating in a situation that you must face almost daily, or even once a week, can be disastrous. It means that, no matter how competently you deal with other situations that threaten your control over your weight, you are repeatedly facing one that you don't know how to deal with. Your frequent failure in this situation keeps pushing you back a step for every step of progress you are making during the rest of the week. You end up playing with the same 5 pounds—losing and gaining, losing and gaining—and you can never reach your goal that way.

To increase your effectiveness in dealing with weight-management problems, we will work with individual situations. So, do the following:

Go back over your ratings for individual situations in the Weight-Mastery Quiz and pencil in two stars by any question that received a confidence rating of 50 percent or less.

Then put one star by questions that received confidence ratings of 55 to 85 percent.

You will use the techniques that I discuss in the next chapter to work on the double-starred situations first, if you have any, and the single-starred situations next.

Our goal is to boost your confidence in all areas of weight management to the 90 percent confidence level or higher. Once you reach the 90 percent confidence level in all of the situations that present weight-management problems, you can feel much more certain that you will be able to manage your weight in the future. And I'm happy to say that it doesn't take *absolute* perfection (which you might have inferred from one of my previous statements above). For example, you will not need to succeed at all times in resisting temptation, but you will need to feel secure that, in the main, you can succeed when you need to. You just need to get from a confidence level of 50 or 60 percent up to 90 percent. Then you will be able to engage in the sort of "controlled bingeing" that poses no threat to your weight.

This is where the candy bar that I give new participants in the Vanderbilt Weight Management Program can play its part in the development of a sense of weight-management mastery. The candy bar is symbolic of all the foods that are difficult to resist right now and that tempt you to make a poor food choice or to overeat.

In the next two chapters I'll show you how you, too, can use a sample of the junk food that ordinarily tempts you to overeat to increase your own sense of weight-management mastery.

10

Four Steps to Mastery: Building Weight-Management Confidence

In order to make the best use of the procedures I am going to describe in this chapter, you really do need to have a candy bar or some other form of junk food right at hand. However, whether or not you have already gone out to purchase that junk food is not as important at this moment as your understanding of why such foods pose a problem for weight management, and how you can learn to deal with them. If, after you read this chapter, you feel that what I have described might be helpful, then you can purchase your candy bar and get to work developing a new and higher level of weight-management confidence.

I want to discuss chocolate as my example because so many persons have trouble dealing with chocolate candy, or other chocolate-flavored dessert foods. And it's no wonder that they do. A chocolate candy bar is not a "normal food"—it's a "supernormal food." It's a scientific blending of the flavors that humans like best. Fat is its primary ingredient (60 percent of the calories in chocolate candy come from fat), followed by sugar, perhaps a pinch of salt to bring out the flavor, and, of course, the chocolate, which, unless blended with fat and sugar, tastes absolutely terrible. It's the creative blending of chocolate with fat and sugar that enables chocolate to work its magic.

Chocolate-flavored foods, as well as other sweet and fatty dessert foods, are designed to turn on appetite even when your hunger has been satisfied. When such foods appear, you begin to salivate, and your pancreas begins to secrete extra insulin in preparation for dealing with the sugar in the food. Both of these reactions actually make you feel hungry, even though you have already eaten. Indeed, every cell in your body seems to turn on all over again and scream, "Eat, eat!"

Candy and most other foods that fall into what is called the "junk-food" category are very hard to resist because of their "supernormal" status. If you have a choice of one of these foods (candy, cake, pie, cookies) or a more natural food, such as fruit, the supernormal food is almost certain to win out. Thus, it becomes very hard for an overweight person to exercise an appropriate choice of foods for weight control when "supernormal" foods are present to compete with normal foods at any given meal or at snacktime.

After I hand out the bar of chocolate to our group of weight-management participants, I ask them whether they can, even in their imagination, see themselves doing exactly what it will take to live with that candy (or whatever food tempts them the most to overeat) and not eat it when it is constantly present in their environments. You might take a moment and do the same thing: can you, in your imagination, see yourself in situations with all of the foods that tempt you the most doing exactly what you are going to need to do for the rest of your life to control your weight?

If you can't even *imagine* yourself doing what you need to do to deal with these situations effectively, how can you ever expect to do it in reality?

Because it is a natural physiological reaction to "turn on" in the presence of "supernormal" foods, the very best strategy for permanent weight management is to control their presence, that is, rarely allow yourself to be in their presence so that you do not have to battle constantly with temptation.

But such control over yourself or your environment is not always possible. I know many of you will have families that bring junk food in unexpectedly, and you may feel that the persons in your family who do not have a problem with their weight should not have to be inconvenienced by your desire to eliminate junk food in the home. Besides, wouldn't it feel great to know that you can control your "bingeing" withou aining weight? Although we normally do not keep quantities of high-calorie foods around the house, right now we have been celebrating the Christmas holidays with visiting house guests and dinner parties. We have one of my wife's incomparable chocolate cheesecakes in the refrigerator, one of my daughter's delicious pumpkin pies right out on the kitchen table, and a quart of my own homemade rum-raisin ice cream in the freezer. (The ice cream is pretty good, too.) Twenty-two years ago I might have overeaten and gained weight with all of these delicious desserts around the house, but not today. I am enjoying these creations— every single one of them—but in moderation. You, too, can learn to enjoy the foods you like best, in quantities that pose no danger for weight control, by practicing the four steps to weight-management mastery.

FOUR STEPS TO WEIGHT-MANAGEMENT MASTERY

You will find it helpful to have one of your own problem areas in mind as I discuss the four steps to weight-management mastery. So, go back over the results of the Weight-Mastery Quiz. Pick out one of the areas in which you have the least confidence in your weight-management ability. This will be the first area of personal concern that you will work on. Keep this problem area in mind to compare with my illustrations as I discuss the techniques.

We use a four-step process to increase your confidence to the maximum. Normally, you will complete all four steps to assure mastery. Because the procedure for gaining confidence and achieving mastery in weight management is very similar to the techniques used by highly accomplished actors, concert musicians, and champion athletes, I am going to use some analogies from these fields to illustrate what I mean.

First, you will need to ask yourself what it is that you need to know and do in order to achieve weight-management mastery in the problem area you have identified. If you don't know what you need to know and do, you can't even take the first step. Sometimes we think we know what we should do to solve a particular weight-management problem, but when we try it, we meet up with unforeseen consequences. In the past, you may have given up in your efforts to change or to control a potential weight-gain situation, but not this time. When you are confronted by unforeseen consequences it simply means that these consequences are your real problems and that you may need some additional skills or knowledge in order to deal with them.

Second, you need to be able to see yourself clearly, in your imagination, carrying out successful weight-management behaviors, just as Olympic champions see themselves performing to perfection in the heat of competition. Champions don't become champions if they imagine themselves failing before they even take to the field!

Third, you may find it helpful to set up rehearsal situations in order to practice what you are learning, just as athletes practice and perfect their skills, in protected, "practice" situations, before they enter their tournaments. (This step is not always possible, and can sometimes be eliminated, but it should be used whenever possible.)

Fourth, you have to expose yourself to the situation that poses the problem and test yourself in reality, just as the athlete does by entering tournaments and competitions. Perhaps you start with those situations that are easiest to handle, and work up to the big time, as musicians and actors do by taking their shows on the road and doing "warm-ups" before hitting Lincoln Center and Broadway.

The relative importance of each of these steps varies with the situation. In addition, as you practice my suggestions, you should expect to develop your own unique approach to using this four-step strategy. My hints will show you how to get started. In the end, you will be your own best weight-management problem-solver.

The methods for dealing with all kinds of food problems, such as resisting temptation and making appropriate food choices, are similar, so I will explain the methods for food-related problems using one illustration. Then I will show you how to apply the four steps to the exercise situation.

A short workbook section is the basis of the next chapter. In this chapter I will show you how to practice our four steps to weight-management mastery in the presence of your choice of junk food. It will help you to reach at least the 90 percent confidence level in dealing with that food. And it will show you how to use the procedure in each of the personally relevant situations on which you have scored below 90 percent confidence in the Weight-Mastery Quiz.

First, some illustrations.

PROBLEM AREAS SUCH AS RESISTING TEMPTATION, SOCIAL EATING, AND POOR FOOD CHOICE

Step 1: Necessary Knowledge and Skills

Most likely you have some idea of what it will take to deal with these problem situations, especially if you have read one of the innumerable behavioral approaches to weight control that are already available, or if you have been in a weight-management program such as Weight Watchers. If you haven't found it possible to implement what you have learned (and, unfortunately, our research shows that over 85 percent of persons who have been in behavioral weight-management programs do not continue to use even one of the control strategies that they learned), these four steps to mastery will help you.

Let's assume that you are in one of the situations described in the Weight-Mastery Quiz. To make it difficult, we will choose a situation that does not permit you to avoid being in the presence of tasty foods.

You are preparing a tasty, full-course dinner.

The question is: what can you do to prevent yourself from snacking during food preparation?

Consider some of the possible strategies. If you have allowed yourself to become overly hungry by skipping meals earlier in the day, do you want to nibble on a free vegetable? If you are not really hungry, but just find that your appetite turns on in the presence of good food, will you chew gum or keep a toothpick in your mouth? Wear a surgical mask? I know some people who wear surgical masks every time they cook a tempting dinner!

Could you just brave it out by imagining how each bite will end up on your hips and keep you in a size 16 or 18 instead of a perfect 10?

I am sure you can think of some additional possibilities for preventing eating at this time. It's up to you to decide what substitute behavior or mental attitude might, with practice, become strong enough to defeat the urge to eat high-calorie foods unnecessarily.

Then you go to Step 2 and do something you have probably neglected to do in the past.

Step 2: Using Fantasy and Your Imagination

Now comes the key—something you have probably never considered doing, nor have you realized its importance. It is being able to see yourself clearly, in your imagination, carrying out your intentions to perfection. I want to elaborate on the importance of this step.

I know that there are many areas in your life in which you are a success. When it comes to performing in these areas, you never think twice—you have no doubt at all about your ability to do what it takes to be successful. If you took a moment to think through what you do in these other areas (even if it is just making a bed, or, at perhaps a more complex level, getting your professional jobs done) you would see yourself in your mind's eye carrying out appropriate acts. But I know that you will have difficulty seeing yourself being this successful with weight-management behaviors, at first.

Having given many concerts in my first career as a violinist, and having become a pretty fair tennis player at a later age, I know what mental work it takes to build self-confidence and then to expose yourself in the arena for the true test of your ability. Actors, musicians, and champion athletes all visualize themselves on the set, the stage, or the field going through the motions that lead to success. We learn to do this as children, and this mental activity is an essential part of practice, just as essential as the physical part. If the actor, musician, or athlete has never learned how to fill his mind with success fantasies, it is quite likely that he will have an anticipation of failure that can become a self-fulfilling prophecy. You may be in this latter situation when it comes to weight management—you expect failure and you get it!

Unfortunately, we tend to forget the role of success fantasies as we grow older. Perhaps we become accustomed to our limitations and, for lack of knowledge or skill, we fail at things, such as controlling our weight, that we could really learn to master. Perhaps we feel sheepish about fantasizing, as though it is not a grown-up thing to do.

It's time to start putting your childhood gift for fantasy and imagination back to work again!

So pick an approach to mastering those eating urges when you are preparing a meal, and take some time out to imagine yourself being completely successful in your performance. It is important to visualize yourself clearly in the situation, actually experiencing the difficulty that you have faced in the past. Then, you visualize yourself going through the specific actions that will lead to mastery, and you boldly carry them out in your mind's eye.

Let me emphasize that *attention to specific behaviors* is very important in this fantasy process. For example, champion tennis players put their major effort into visualizing perfect strokes and their plan of attack. They spend much less time dreaming of the trophy! This is where most persons who attempt to use fantasy as an aid to change make their crucial mistake. They dream about the end product, whereas they should be concentrating on the *means* to that end. As a concert violinist it was one thing to dream about being a success on the stage, but I soon learned that the most profitable time had to be spent mentally rehearsing the bowings and fingerings of every selection I was to perform, and hearing the music I was working on in my mind's ear as I watched the score flow by my closed eyes. Working mentally with a great deal of attention to detail, I was able to increase my technical security and I never had a memory slip.

You, too, will build confidence in the technique as you practice, and as you continue with the next steps in the mastery process. And, by the way, the time when you are out walking alone, or engaging in any other solitary physical activity, is one of the best times for productive fantasy. That's when you can engage in the mental practice that is necessary to learning to control your weight. Soon you may find that you are applying mental practice or rehearsal to many other things in your life. Today, being alone in some physical activity has become my best time for mental practice, and it makes going for a jog in the woods my best time for preparing classes and speeches and outlining articles and books. Try it—being alone during a walk or a job may become your most productive and creative time as well.

Step 3: Setting Up a Rehearsal Situation

Before you put yourself to a major test, it is always good to practice in one that minimizes the difficulties so that you can build your skills.

In the food-preparation situation, practice making a small meal, or preparing only one simple dish. In addition, begin with practice at a time when the temptations to eat inappropriately are slight. Making breakfast, lunch, or a snack is a good time. After going through what is required in your imagination, set up your kitchen in a way that will minimize the temptation to nibble (don't have a large array of particularly tempting foods around), make your meal, carry it to the table, and sit down to eat in accordance with your plan. Review what you did (and did *not* do), and get it firmly established in your mind so that, if asked, you could repeat every detail accurately.

One of the best ways to build up your strength to resist eating in this situation (and in others that I will describe in a moment) is to invite a friend over to observe you as you demonstrate your procedures for gaining control. Explain what you are about to do and imagine that your friend is your coach. Then, practice in front of your coach.

And don't forget to give yourself some credit for success. Have you ever seen the raised fist of the champion tennis player after a great shot? You need to do a little of the same as you accumulate your weight-management victories.

Step 4: Exposing Yourself to the Real Test

After a few successes in your rehearsal situations, you are ready for the real thing. Before you try it, see yourself as a success in your imagination, going through the entire process from beginning to end. And, as in rehearsal, it may prove helpful to invite someone in to watch, explaining beforehand what you are about to do. Public commitment helps increase the incentive to succeed. For example, continuing with the food-preparation situation, announce that tonight is the night for putting your approach to preventing nibbling to work. Then, invite members of the family to drop by to observe you, acting like a weight-management champion. And invite *them* to be your food tasters!

Additional Examples for Other Eating Situations

As I indicated, you must become your own best problem-solver, but I might be able to assist with some other hints.

In the category of *resisting temptation*, when you feel the urge to eat in the evening, or on weekends when you have nothing else pressing to do for a few moments, or when those snack foods are likely to pop up in front of you as you watch TV, it is good to have some alternative activity available to replace eating, or a substitute food that you have practiced turning to in your imagination and rehearsal. We practice saying "No, thanks" in our groups when we work on *social eating* situations. First we use our imagination and then we rehearse and role-play with real, tempting high-calorie foods that I bring to the group meetings for this special purpose. Then we send our participants home to set up practice situations.

With *food choice*, you might imagine that cake and fruit are both available as desserts, either at home or in a restaurant. Then, fantasize yourself executing the behavior you desire for weight control. Get closer to reality by actually buying yourself that symbolic candy bar; set it out on a table together with a piece of any kind of fresh fruit that you like, pick up the fruit and put the candy away (it is better out of sight!), and eat your fruit.

The food-choice situation is one that is helped by mentally rehearsing the rewards of a correct choice. These rewards are often postponed to the future and they are not as naturally strong as the taste of cake, cookies, or candy. Although a correct choice of fruit over junk food would either get you closer to your weight goal, keep you at desirable weight, or simply help you stay healthier than the candy, a "supernormal" food is a very strong physiological stimulus to eating. If it is present right in front of you, it can overwhelm all other considerations—that is, unless you put thoughts of future consequences right at the forefront of your consciousness, and then move with dispatch to a correct choice.

Finally, with *overeating*, most of us have the urge to throw in the towel the moment we make the first deviation from our eating vows. It is very important that you begin to see yourself in a different light. Yes, it is possible to *begin* to overeat, and *still stop yourself*. Work through the familiar fantasy steps that you have used in the other eating problem areas: imagine yourself beginning to overeat, and then exerting control. It is most important that you see yourself returning immediately to your eating and activity program, so that one skirmish lost does not lead to losing the entire war.

One of the best rehearsal strategies for learning to deal with overeating is to buy a food item that frequently tempts you to overeat, in a single portion, and set up a situation in which you can eat it slowly and with pleasure. It helps to do things like this before an audience as you talk through what you are experiencing and doing—so invite a friend to be with you as you practice. Be sure to allow up to twenty minutes for observing yourself and your reactions after you finish eating, so that you can see how your appetite begins to turn off and how the urge to continue disappears. Then store the image of the experience in your memory so you can draw on it as needed.

MAINTAINING YOUR EXERCISE PROGRAM

What do you need to do when every bone in your body seems to say it would be so much more pleasant to sit down after a hard day, with a snack at your side, rather than go for a walk?

What can you do to deal with a feeling of fatigue when the feeling, in fact, doesn't result from physical exertion? When, instead, it is more mental than physical?

How will you deal with the demands of daily living when each and every one of them begins to seem like it is more important than taking that walk or going to your dance class?

Step 1: Choosing the Strategies That Can Lead to Success

As I have said in a previous chapter, nothing proves to be a greater remedy for fatigue and sluggish feelings than the very physical activity you have the urge to resist. Once you have become an active person, you will still have a resistance to exercise at odd times, but you will be able to envision the refreshing and relaxing feelings that follow activity. Getting this anticipatory feeling up front in your imagination can become all the incentive you need to get started.

In addition, learning to say no to outside demands and putting your health priorities at their deserved levels, for just forty-five minutes or so a day, are, in my opinion, inalienable rights! I think you, too, should cultivate this attitude and then consider what it will take to negotiate with others to obtain the time and support.

Step 2: Using Fantasy and Your Imagination

You start by imagining that one of the situations has occurred, for example, a fatigue situation, and that you have developed a plan. You then imagine how you will feel when you are really, really tired and resistant, but know that the feelings are from frustrations you encountered at work or that they result simply from the stress of being forced to work sitting down all day. (The sitting position, when it is necessary for most of your workday, causes a significant amount of physical stress, especially to the lower back and shoulders, and leads to a great deal of fatigue.) Then, clearly see yourself overcoming these resistant feelings and setting out for a walk. Just imagine how it will feel to get out of the house and take a breath of fresh air. Or imagine how it will feel when no one knows where you are and cannot bother you for forty-five minutes. Imagine the feeling you will have when you finish—both physical and mental. And, once again, in your imagination, give yourself the congratulations you deserve for having been able to accomplish a most important weight-management activity.

Step 3: Rehearsal

The practice behavior I am about to suggest may seem paradoxical, but it works very well in developing an amazing amount of control over your feelings. It has, in fact, been used as a therapeutic procedure with top flight athletes who were having trouble performing at their peak levels.

The next time you are about to go for a walk, or engage in any other physical activity, hesitate for just a moment before you begin. Now, even though you are feeling full of energy, imagine instead that you are feeling very tired and not at all in the mood for activity. Go ahead and do it—turn on your very *worst* feelings. Then, after just a few moments, turn on your energy and begin your exercise with vigor. You will find that you have a great deal of ability to switch your feelings on and off. Switch back and forth, and see how it feels. Then, the next time you feel tired and sluggish, turn on your vigor switch, get moving, and in moments you will feel truly invigorated.

Similarly, if you have problems negotiating for personal time, imagine and rehearse what it will take to bargain for what you need with your family or with your boss. I know some very busy (and very successful) people who felt that they had to work incessantly. They had luncheon meetings and after-work business cocktail meetings every day, and they carried their briefcases home loaded with work every night. If you are in the same circumstances, your first step is to imagine that change is possible, followed by a little rehearsal, which might include talking over a strategy for changing the situation with a friend or business associate.

Step 4: Testing Yourself in the Real Situation

After you have gone through the steps above, you are ready for the real test. You now have a good strategy for dealing with fatigue. Use it and you will achieve virtual perfection in handling all fatigue problems (but remember not to force yourself into activity when you are ill, especially when you have a fever).

When it comes to negotiating for personal time, most of the persons I have worked with have found that they themselves were their own worst enemies. You don't have to work every waking hour, and you can get the cooperation of your family if you approach family responsibilities as a family sharing proposition. Begin with the attitude that you will cooperate with others so that they can get what they need in order to lead happy and fulfilling lives, and that they, in turn, owe you help in getting forty-five minutes for yourself and your health.

Best of all, you are more than likely to discover that an activity break, even a brief one, at some point during your actual working hours will lead to greater productivity and job satisfaction. It works so well that some corporations are beginning to make activity breaks a required part of the working day. Why not work fewer hours, get more done, and enjoy your work more, all at the same time? If you cannot manage longer periods of time, at least experiment with some fifteen-minute work breaks. You may have to force yourself to take these breaks at first. But after a while you may be quite surprised at the results, in both productivity and good feelings.

A NOTE ON JUNK FOOD

Before you begin to use the workbook and the four steps to weight-management mastery, I think you will be able to raise your weight) than it does of the Recommended Dietary Allow-understand what a junk food really is.

A "junk food" is a food that supplies a larger percentage of your total daily need for calories (the amount it takes to maintain your weight) than it does of the Recommended Dietary Allowance of any single essential vitamin or mineral.

Read some food labels and you will see exactly what I mean. For example, take the label from a chocolate bar. It is a 1.45-ounce bar, which you can pick up at any grocery. The label says that it contains 230 calories. If you are a woman who needs about 1800 calories a day to maintain your weight at the present time, 230 calories is almost 13 percent (it is actually 12.7 percent) of the calories you need to maintain your weight. However, the most that this chocolate bar contains of any one essential vitamin or mineral is just 8 percent of the Recommended Dietary Allowance of calcium (because of the milk content). In other words, junk foods contain relatively more weight-maintaining calories than they do health-sustaining essential nutrients such as vitamins and minerals.

If you will think about it for just a minute, I think you will see that, if your diet is composed of a large extent of junk foods, you will reach (or go beyond) your required number of weight-maintenance calories *but you will still be undernourished in terms of essential vitamins and minerals*. Although I cannot prove this point, I think another reason that many persons may be stimulated to overeat when their diets contain many junk foods is that their bodies are pushing them to take in enough food to meet its nutritional needs in vitamins and minerals.

A serving of a truly nourishing food contains a larger percentage of at least three or four of the essential vitamins and minerals—those nutrients you need to maintain health and fitness—than it does of your total daily need for calories.

Now consider how you can ruin a perfectly nourishing food. Take a potato, for example. A 3½-ounce baked potato contains about 90 calories (compared with the 230 calories in just 1.45 ounces of milk chocolate). Ninety calories is only 5 percent of the total calories that it takes to maintain your weight (at 1800 calories per day). But that 3½-ounce baked potato *is a powerhouse when it comes to nourishment*. For each 5 percent of your total daily calories, it contains (based on Recommended Dietary Allowances) approximately:

  7 percent of your daily protein needs
  8 percent of your phosphorus needs
  10 percent of your thiamine needs
  13 percent of your niacin needs
  33 percent of your vitamin C needs
  plus about 25 percent of the suggested minimum for potassium, and a broad array of traces of other vitamins and minerals. (That potassium content makes it excellent for helping to prevent water retention, since the potato contains almost no sodium and a high potassium-to-sodium ratio helps the kidneys eliminate excess water from the system.)

Now, look what happens when you peel and fry up these otherwise nutritious potatoes and convert them to french fries: a similar 3½-ounce serving will add up to approximately *275 calories!* You have added over 180 calories' worth of fat! And you will have almost succeeded in converting that poor potato into a junk food. In a 90-calorie serving (that's less than 1.2 ounces, or just about three or four little strips, rather than a whole baked potato), you will obtain only:

  3.5 percent of your daily protein needs
  4.6 percent of your phosphorus needs
  4 percent of your thiamine needs
  7.7 percent of your niacin needs
  11 percent of your vitamin C needs
  and only about 11 percent of the suggested minimum for potassium.

In just about every way, except for fat calories, you have cut the nutritional value of a potato by about two-thirds when you eat french fries. EVERY TIME THAT YOU EAT FRIED FOODS, THIS IS WHAT YOU ARE DOING: YOU ARE TRIPLING THE CALORIES PER SERVING, OR, FOR EQUAL CALO-RIE SERVINGS, YOU ARE CUTTING THE OTHER NUTRI-TIONAL VALUE OF YOUR FOOD BY ABOUT TWO-THIRDS!

Begin to read some of the labels on those foods that tempt you to overeat. Check out all dessert and snack foods, including salty, rather than sweet, snacks. You will see that, in just about every case, they contain a larger percentage of your total daily calorie needs than they contain of even *one* vitamin or mineral. By eating a large amount of junk food, you may be keeping yourself fat *and malnourished* at the same time!

Because we vary in our daily need for calories at mainte-nance levels, I suggest you use the following rule of thumb for determining whether a food falls into the "junk" category: Examine the label and simply calculate whether it contains 5 percent of the RDA of at least one vitamin or mineral for every 100 calories. Thus, if a serving of some snack, according to the label of the package, is 100 calories, it ought to have 5 percent of at least one essential vitamin or mineral listed; if a serving is 200 calories, it ought to have 10 percent of at least one vitamin or mineral.

Really nutritious foods that you can use as snacks, such as the grapefruit that I used as my safe fruit, have a much higher percentage of essential vitamins and minerals than they do of your weight-maintenance calories. For example, 100 calories' worth of grapefruit (I prefer pink varieties) contains 7 percent of the RDA for iron, 22 percent of vitamin A, 12 percent of thiamine, 5 percent of riboflavin, 5 percent of niacin, 192 percent of vitamin C, and about 14 percent of potassium. And since grapefruit contains virtually no sodium, that high potassi-um content makes it an excellent food for persons who tend to retain water.

If you have difficulty making good food choices, I hope these words will increase your motivation to reduce permanently the junk food in your diet and to begin to make more nutritious substitutions for snacks and desserts. I also hope that I have motivated you to make some of the other changes I suggest, such as increasing your activity level if you are a sedentary person. If so, I think using the workbook for the four steps to weight-management mastery, which I present in the next chapter, will help you maintain the initiatives you have taken in beginning the Rotation Diet.

11

A Weight-Mastery Workbook

I know you are going to be reluctant to do this, especially after my discussion of junk food at the end of the previous chapter, but you have to go to the grocery and buy a candy bar, or a bag of chocolate chip cookies, or whatever other junk food that has, in the past, been a part of your weight-management problem. Pick your most-difficult-to-deal-with junk food!

But before you purchase your junk food, rate yourself on the following question, just as you did on the Weight-Mastery Quiz in Chapter 9:

> You have enough of your favorite junk food in the house to last you (and your family) a month. How confident are you that you will be able to live with that junk food for a full month and not eat any? Let me phrase the question another way: *What is the probability that you will be able to keep that food in the house for a full month and not eat any?*
>
> Your rating: _____

How did you rate yourself? Zero percent? Fifty percent? From now on, after you complete the first exercise I am about to describe, this will all be different.

After you use the four steps to weight-management mastery

and the junk food that you will purchase as your tool and your symbol, you are going to have a completely different relationship with junk food. You are going to end up at least 90 percent confident in your ability to manage your appetite for such foods.

An increase in your confidence to deal with junk food can have a tremendous impact for the better on your ability to control your weight, because, if you are anything like the persons in the Vanderbilt Weight Management Program, the increase in rated confidence is closely translated into action. Suppose you have just rated yourself at the 50 percent confidence level. An increase to 90 percent confidence means that you will be successful in resisting junk food (if you choose to) four out of five times that you might prevously have eaten some (or more than "some").

Let me remind you once again that we are not after abstinence. We are aiming for an increase in control to the point where you can decide, with great confidence, on when and where it will be time for a "controlled binge."

For this first exercise to be of maximum value to you, you must not use any junk foods that you already have in the house. You must use some food that is especially purchased for this exercise, so that you can clearly see the role that your state of mind can play in controlling your eating temptations. This will become clear to you as you go through the exercise in a way that cannot be communicated through reading about it. So, make a special trip and buy your special, "symbolic" junk food. Trust me—take my word that it is best if you do it this way, and do it!

HOW TO USE YOUR SPECIAL JUNK FOOD AS A TOOL AND A SYMBOL OF YOUR ABILITY TO DEAL WITH TEMPTATION

Step 1: What Would You Need to Do If You Were to Succeed in Not Eating This Food during the Next Month?

Perhaps the first thing that occurs to you is to not buy it in the first place! Avoiding temptation is a number one strategy and one worth using as a matter of course, considering the natural physiological reactions to the sight of "supernormal" foods. But not buying the food or giving it away (which many of our participants in the Vanderbilt Weight Management Program suggest as a means of avoiding temptation) would defeat the purpose of the exercise. Your objective is to increase your ability to have junk foods in your immediate environment and not eat them in amounts that would lead to a weight gain.

In the space below, list the things that you might possibly do that would prevent you from eating this food during the next month. Here are a few suggestions that we discuss in our weight-management groups:

Hide it—get it out of sight.

Wrap it in "plain brown paper" and stick it in the freezer.

Put it out in plain sight and practice sitting next to it without eating it.

Review carefully the effects the overindulgence in junk food will have on your weight.

Think about the effects that not eating it and substituting a more nutritious food will have on your weight and your health.

Think about how you feel after you eat junk food and how much more positive you will feel about yourself if you don't, or if you eat only a planned amount.

Think about using it in a "controlled binge" after you finish twenty-one days on the Rotation Diet.

What do you think will work for you? (It helps to write down your thoughts about potential strategies.)

_____

_____

_____

Step 2: Use Your Imagination in Mental Rehearsal

This is a key step that many people, otherwise well versed in all the behavioral eating-control strategies, fail to use. Before you attempt to implement any strategy that might help you control your inclination to eat this junk food during the next month, go through the entire process involved in implementing your approach very carefully in your imagination. See the process through in great detail from beginning to end. Experience the difficulties in your fantasy, if you anticipate any, but, by all means, see yourself as being ultimately successful, and celebrate that success in your imagination.

Be sure to visualize yourself as being in the presence of this food, at least for some certain limited time, before you imagine yourself getting it out of sight, and see yourself successfully resisting any urge to eat it. Feel the urge, if you anticipate any, but visualize yourself doing whatever it will take not to eat any.

Then, as part of another scene, try visualizing yourself eating your junk food at a time when you have planned to include some such foods in your diet, for example, after three weeks on the Rotation Diet. If you are at all like me, I suspect that you will want to enjoy some dessert foods at appropriate times, without losing control. So, it is valuable to work such situations into your mental rehearsal.

Step 3: Physical Rehearsal and Practice

After you have had a session or two of mental practice in which you have planned how you will deal with your junk food, do it in reality. Do exactly what you have been rehearsing in your fantasy. This is another instance in which it can help to have an audience, or to announce your intention publicly, and then do it! Even if it all sounds crazy to your friends, you will increase your ability to deal with junk food if you talk about what you are doing with other people, and if you illustrate what you are doing in reality.

And remember that one of the most important things you can do, when junk food is not in your food plan, is to be able to say, unequivocally, "No, thanks" when someone offers you some junk food. Using the junk food you have purchased as a prop, have a friend offer it to you and practice saying "No, thanks" until it becomes automatic—at least as easy to say as, "Well, I really shouldn't—" as you used to say, when you previously reached for the junk food and were about to "blow it."

Step 4: Testing Yourself in the Real World

BEFORE GOING ON TO THIS STEP, REPEAT THE QUES-
TION TO YOURSELF THAT I INTRODUCED AT THE
BEGINNING OF THIS CHAPTER IN THIS SLIGHTLY
MODIFIED FORM: How confident are you that you can be in
the physical presence of your symbolic junk food, or any other
tempting junk food, and not eat it?

You are ready for the real-world test when you can answer
that question with a 90 percent level of confidence.

Keep repeating Steps 1 to 3 until you reach at least a 90
percent confidence level.

Then, put yourself in the line of fire intentionally. Plan to
go out with family or friends to any party or restaurant where
junk food is a standard part of the menu, or put yourself in the
presence of junk food in any convenient way, such as going to a
dessert shop or ice cream parlor. Have your rehearsed strategies
clearly in your mind. See if you can plan a situation with
minimal temptation at first. However, if you have worked through
the other three steps, you will probably be able to deal with just
about any junk food temptation.

When you have worked through this exercise with your
symbolic junk food, I think you will see why I wanted you to
purchase it specially. From now on, every time you purchase
any sort of food that previously incited you to overeat, you will
purchase it in the frame of mind you have cultivated with your
symbolic food. I think you will find that you have developed
something that, in the past, you might have called *willpower*. But
you will also find that controlling your appetite for such foods
will not feel like the struggle you might have associated with that
word. You now have a new, and well-practiced, repertoire of
responses for resisting junk-food temptations and making better
food choices.

USING THE FOUR STEPS TO WEIGHT-MANAGEMENT MASTERY IN YOUR OWN MOST RELEVANT SITUATIONS

So much for the junk food practice. Now let's get on with one of your own double-starred situations (or single-starred situations if you do not have any marked with double stars).

Go back to the Weight-Mastery Quiz and choose one of your least confident scenes. In the space below, rewrite the scene so that it is an accurate representation of what you actually face. Describe the scene in whatever detail is necessary for completeness—who is there, what the room looks like, how it feels, etc. The more detailed and complete, the better.

_____
_____
_____
_____
_____
_____
_____
_____
_____

Before going any further, consider once again how confident you are that you can carry out an appropriate weight-management behavior in this situation and write it down, in the space below.

Confidence rating in your ability to carry out an appropriate weight-management behavior in the above situation is _____ .

Now you are ready to lead yourself in the four-step plan to weight-management mastery.

Step 1: Write Down All of the Things That Occur to You That Might Help You Deal Successfully with This Situation

If you have trouble developing a plan of action, reread the last two chapters for some hints.

_____
_____
_____
_____

Step 2: Practice Your Solutions in Your Imagination

See yourself performing in exactly the way it will take to be a complete success. Remember, it's the *means* to success that you must mentally rehearse—each and every step—and this is different from "dreaming" about being successful. Take time to work on it, every day if necessary. We tell participants in the Vanderbilt groups to spend at least five minutes a day for a week, if necessary. And, interestingly enough, just five minutes a day seems to be enough.

Step 3: Set Up a Practice Situation

Insofar as is possible, set up some physical rehearsals or practice sessions. This step is not always possible, but, use my musician, actor, and sports analogies of Chapter 10 (pages 160–161) to help you design whatever warm-ups you can think of.

Step 4: Test Yourself in the Real World

Before going on to Step 4, ask yourself the confidence question once again to determine whether you have reached the 90 percent level. That's the time to proceed with the real-world test. Keep everything you have been working on in the forefront of your consciousness as you intentionally subject yourself to the troublesome situation.

DEALING WITH THE UNFORESEEN CONSEQUENCES OF CHANGE

The moment you try to change anything about yourself or your dealings with other people, something unforeseen happens. You may fail to be able to carry out your practiced intentions because you have not correctly identified the problem!

Think about this for a moment: the things that happen to you as you go about making changes, that prevent you from carrying out your intentions, are what constitute your real problems. I will give two examples.

A simple one first, to illustrate the point: you eat too fast and you are told that it is helpful to slow down by putting your fork down between bites, or for two minutes in the middle of a meal. You put the fork down and then what happens? You don't know what to do with your hands; you don't know what to say to the folks around you who are staring at you; you get very fidgety waiting for two minutes to pass. What's the real problem? It's learning to deal with what happens after you put the fork down!

A more difficult one: you are a woman and agree with me that you have a right to forty-five minutes a day of exercise for your personal well-being and you rehearse what you will say to your mate to negotiate for this time. He agrees in principle, but he pouts or acts surly every time it is his turn to take over the family responsibilities to help you accomplish your objectives. This upsets you and leads to an argument. Your problem is not knowing how to deal with a pouting, surly husband.

When unforeseen consequences arise as a result of your efforts to make changes, DON'T ACCEPT DEFEAT. Just redefine the problem and put it back into my four-step weight-mastery procedure. Think about possible solutions to these unforeseen consequences, go through the three preliminary steps before attempting to deal with the situation in reality, and TRY AGAIN— AND AGAIN, if necessary.

And keep telling yourself one indisputable fact: the difference between successful people and unsuccessful people is that successful people never give up!

12

Alternate Menus for the Rotation Diet

I asked our nutrition consultant to the Vanderbilt Weight Management Program, Ms. Rachel Willis, R.D., to design some alternate menus for the Rotation Diet to show you the interest and variety that you can add to a healthful weight-reduction and weight-maintenance diet. Except for breakfasts, which are often the same, I asked her to be as different as possible from the standard menus in the design of the meals and in her style of cooking, and, of course, to maximize the nutritional value of the food selections at every calorie level of the Rotation Diet plan. She has come up with some great recipes, illustrating styles of food preparation from all over the world, while using tricks for saving calories and enhancing flavors in everything from soups and salads to main courses and some great desserts.

You can choose a complete day from the Alternate Menus to substitute for any equivalent day in the standard menus on your second time around (Week 3) on the Rotation Diet. Just make sure you are at the appropriate calorie level. I include several days at each level of the Rotation Diet, from 600 to 1800 calories, among the Alternate Menus.

If you do not feel like sticking with any full day in its entirety, you can mix and match your own meals. The calories are listed for all recipes in this chapter, as well as for the standard recipes in Chapter 6. Choose a standard breakfast at each level, if you like, and repeat it for several days if that will make your food choice easier. (If you choose a fortified cereal for breakfast, such as 40% Bran Flakes or Raisin Bran, you will help ensure that the nutritional value of your diet closely approximates the RDA's, even at 600 calories per day.)

For lunch and dinner, however, be sure to include a wide variety of different foods both during your twenty-one days on the Rotation Diet and in maintenance.

If you design your own menus at any time during the Rotation Diet, remember the formula:

WOMEN— *For Weeks 1 and 3:*
600 calories for three days
900 calories for four days
For Week 2:
1200 calories for one week

MEN— *For Weeks 1 and 3:*
1200 calories for three days
1500 calories for four days
For Week 2:
1800 calories for one week

MAINTENANCE

Women

The 1500- and 1800-calorie menus in this chapter are perfect for women as you build up to your maintenance intake after the Rotation Diet. Try them to ensure that you do not regain any weight. You can alternate these menus, or substitute them, for the 1500- and 1800-calorie-per-day menus that I suggest for men in Chapter 6. If you wish to follow your own inclinations on your way to maintenance, be sure to increase by only 300 calories per day, and stick with 1500 for several days before going up to 1800.

Men

On entering maintenance, men should also remember to increase from 1800 calories per day, up to your maintenance levels, in amounts of about 300 calories per day. Be sure to stay with 2100 calories per day for several days, checking your weight, before moving up to 2400. It is best to increase your calories with fruits, vegetables, whole grains, and lean meats, but you can try a serving of a dessert or alcoholic beverage if you like. Check my quick calorie guide in Appendix A to make sure you do not increase by too much too rapidly.

Everyone

Remember that *free vegetables* and your *safe fruit* are available at all times, and that a substitution of fruit of any kind for junk-food snacks will go a long way toward preventing weight gain after you have used the Rotation Diet to reach your goal.

MEAL PREPARATION WITH THE ALTERNATE MENUS

Any of the dishes marked by an asterisk in the Alternate Menus that follow will have a recipe in this chapter, right after the daily menu plans. Some of the dishes from the standard menus have been included, so if you do not see an asterisk after a dish in the Alternate Menus, be sure to check the index or go directly to Chapter 6 to find some cooking suggestions. If you follow your own inclinations, remember to prepare food in a plain fashion, without added fat or sugar, except as permitted in each rotation. All weights in the following menus are cooked weights. The calorie counts in the recipes allow for shrinkage due to cooking.

600-Calorie Rotation

MENU 1

Breakfast

½ grapefruit
½ cup of oatmeal
½ teaspoon of cinnamon
4 ounces of skim milk
Coffee or tea

Lunch

1 cup of bouillon
Open-faced sandwich: 1 slice of whole-grain bread,
1 ounce of lean meat, and Dijon mustard
Unlimited free vegetables
No-Cal Salad Dressing
½ cup of peach slices
4 ounces of skim milk
No-cal beverage

Dinner

2 ounces of veal cutlet, pan- or oven-broiled
Fresh spinach salad
No-Cal Salad Dressing
½ cup of brown rice
No-cal beverage

MENU 2

Breakfast

8 ounces of plain yogurt
1 cup of berries, sliced
1 slice of whole-grain toast
Coffee or tea

Lunch

Chef salad: add 1 ounce of turkey, carrots, bell
peppers, celery, and unlimited free vegetables
No-Cal Salad Dressing
5 whole-wheat crackers
No-cal beverage

Dinner

1 cup of red beans
½ cup of brown rice
2 tablespoons of grated cheese
½ cup of cauliflower
½ grapefruit
No-cal beverage

MENU **3**

Breakfast

Cheese toast: 1 ounce of cheese and
1 slice of whole-grain bread
1 orange
Coffee or tea

Lunch

Tomato stuffed with ¼ cup of shrimp or tuna
1 cup of tossed salad
No-Cal Salad Dressing
5 whole-wheat crackers
1 apple
No-cal beverage

Dinner

Egg Drop Soup*
Turkey and sprout sandwich: open-faced with 1 slice of whole-grain bread, 1 ounce of turkey, and Dijon mustard
¼ cantaloupe
No-cal beverage

900-Calorie Rotation

MENU 1

Breakfast

1 low-fat Whole-Wheat Breakfast Cake*
2 tablespoons of maple syrup
8 ounces of skim milk
Choice of fruit
Coffee or tea

Lunch

2 ounces of Baked Chicken
1 cup of Spinach Salad
No-Cal or Lo-Cal Salad Dressing
½ cup of fresh fruit
No-cal beverage

Dinner

3 ounces of Seafood Italia*
½ cup of cooked carrots
1 cup of Herb and Garlic Brussels Sprouts*
1 baked potato
1 teaspoon of butter or 2 teaspoons of sour cream
No-cal beverage

MENU 2

Breakfast

8 ounces of skim milk
½ cup of hot cereal
½ teaspoon of cinnamon
2 tablespoons of raisins
Coffee or tea

Lunch

Cup of soup (your choice)
Open-faced sandwich: 1 slice of whole-grain bread
with 2 ounces of lean meat, sliced tomato,
and Dijon mustard
1 cup of lettuce salad with carrots, celery,
and cucumber
No-Cal or Lo-Cal Salad Dressing
½ grapefruit
No-cal beverage

Dinner

2 ounces of Chicken Sesame*
¾ cup of brown rice
¾ cup of yellow squash
1 cup of fresh fruit
No-cal beverage

MENU 3

Breakfast

1 ounce of dry cereal
4 ounces of skim milk

1 orange
Coffee or tea

Lunch

4 ounces of Medley Casserole*
½ cup of Peas and Pods*
4 ounces of skim milk
½ grapefruit
No-cal beverage

Dinner

3 ounces of Paprika Pork Goulash*
½ cup of noodles
1 cup of broccoli
1 pear or peach
No-cal beverage

MENU 4

Breakfast

½ cup of cooked cereal
2 tablespoons of raisins
8 ounces of skim milk
Coffee or tea

Lunch

1 cup of bouillon
1 roll of Rolled Ham and Vegetables*
1 cup of tossed salad
No-Cal or Lo-Cal Salad Dressing
5 whole-wheat crackers
1 apple
No-cal beverage

Dinner

4 ounces of Chicken Divan*
1 baked potato
1 teaspoon of butter or 2 teaspoons of sour cream
½ cup of cauliflower
1 cup of berries and melon balls
No-cal beverage

1200-Calorie Rotation

Remember that when you reach the 1200-calorie level, or above, you may add 1 tablespoon of butter, oil, or other fat within the calorie guidelines. You may also add 3 *safe fruits* within the calorie guidelines.

MENU **1**

Breakfast

8 ounces of skim milk
½ banana
1¼ cup of dry cereal
Coffee or tea

Lunch

1 cup of salad: lettuce, tomato, radish, green pepper
Lo-Cal Salad Dressing
6 whole-wheat crackers
8 ounces of plain yogurt
1 cup of berries
No-cal beverage

Dinner

4 ounces of Baked Fish in Spring Herbs*
1 cup of Oven-fried Potatoes*
1 cup of cooked cabbage
1 apple
No-cal beverage

MENU **2**

Breakfast

8 ounces of skim milk
½ cup of oatmeal with cinnamon
2 tablespoons of raisins
1 slice of whole-grain toast
Coffee or tea

Lunch

1 cup of Broccoli-Cauliflower Soup*
5 whole-wheat crackers
1 ounce of cheddar cheese
1 cup of tossed salad
Lo-Cal Salad Dressing
½ grapefruit
No-cal beverage

Dinner

3 ounces of Veal in Mushroom Sauce*
1 cup of steamed asparagus
1 cup of boiled new potatoes
1 cup of fresh fruit
1 slice of whole-grain bread
No-cal beverage

Breakfast

8 ounces of plain yogurt
1 cup of berries and melon balls
1 slice of whole-wheat toast
Coffee or tea

Lunch

12 ounces of Mushroom Clam Chowder*
1 cup of Seasoned Tomato Salad*
4 Toasted Oat Thins*
½ grapefruit
No-cal beverage

Dinner

4 ounces of Halibut Steak with Vegetables*
1 cup of Carrots Aloha*
¾ cup of Peas and Baby Onions
1 cup of sliced peaches
No-cal beverage

MENU 4

Breakfast

8 ounces of skim milk
1 low-fat Whole-Wheat Breakfast Cake*
2 tablespoons of maple syrup
½ banana
Coffee or tea

Lunch

1 cup of Egg Drop Soup*
Chicken and Swiss Salad*
½ melon
No-cal beverage

Dinner

4 ounces of Spicy Orange Pork*
1 cup of Herb and Garlic Brussels Sprouts*
½ cup of brown rice
½ cup of unsweetened applesauce
1 cup of tossed greens
Lo-Cal Salad Dressing
No-cal beverage

MENU 5

Breakfast

8 ounces of skim milk
1 German Fruit Puff*
Coffee or tea

Lunch

1 serving of Cheddar Chili Pie*
Unlimited free vegetables
Lo-Cal Salad Dressing
6 whole-wheat crackers
1 pear
No-cal beverage

Dinner

4 ounces of Chicken Teriyaki*
1 serving of Chinese Fried Rice*
1 cup of steamed zucchini
1 serving of Honeydew De-Light*
No-cal beverage

MENU 6

Breakfast

8 ounces of skim milk
1 slice of whole-wheat toast
1 teaspoon of preserves
1 orange
Coffee or tea

Lunch

1 cup of soup (your choice)
2 slices of whole-grain bread
2 ounces of chicken
Unlimited free vegetables
Lo-Cal Salad Dressing
½ melon
No-cal beverage

Dinner

4 ounces of lean broiled beefsteak
1 cup of brown rice
1 cup of green beans
1 cup of peach slices
No-cal beverage

MENU 7

Breakfast

4 ounces of skim milk
1 bagel
½ grapefruit
Coffee or tea

Lunch

Turkey and sprout sandwich: open-faced with 1
slice of whole-grain bread, 1 ounce of turkey,
and Dijon mustard
1 cup of Spinach Caesar Salad*
1 banana
1 cup of bouillon
No-cal beverage

Dinner

4 ounces of Chicken Cordon Bleu*
1 cup of Spicy Green Beans*
1 small baked potato
1 slice of Tropical Coconut Crust Pie*
No-cal beverage

1500-Calorie Rotation

MENU 1

Breakfast

8 ounces of skim or low-fat milk
1 cup of hot cereal
2 tablespoons of raisins
4 ounces of grapefruit juice
Coffee or tea

Lunch

10 ounces of Veal Stew*
5 whole-wheat crackers
1 apple
No-cal beverage

Dinner

4 ounces of Chicken Oahu*
1 cup of steamed broccoli
½ cup of Island Rice*
2 Chewy Raisin Cookies*
No-cal beverage

MENU 2

Breakfast

1½ ounces of dry cereal
1 banana
8 ounces of skim or low-fat milk
Coffee or tea

Lunch

¾ cup of cottage cheese
6 whole-wheat crackers
1 cup of steamed cauliflower
½ melon
No-cal beverage

Dinner

12 ounces of Shrimp Jambalaya*
1 cup of Green Beans and Mushrooms*
1 cup of cooked carrots
5 whole wheat-crackers
1 slice of Tropical Coconut Crust Pie*
No-cal beverage

MENU 3

Breakfast

8 ounces of plain yogurt
1 cup of berries
1 slice of whole-wheat toast
Coffee or tea

Lunch

1 cup of soup (your choice)
2 slices of whole-grain bread
¼ cup of Tuna Salad
Unlimited free vegetables
Lo-Cal Salad Dressing
1 banana
No-cal beverage

Dinner

One-fourth Lean and Perfect Pizza*
1½ cups of tossed salad
Lo-Cal Salad Dressing
1 cup of fruit
No-cal beverage

MENU **4**

Breakfast

8 ounces of skim or low-fat milk
1 German Fruit Puff*
Coffee or tea

Lunch

4 ounces of Quick Skillet*
1 cup of tossed greens
Lo-Cal Salad Dressing
1 apple
No-cal beverage

Dinner

4 ounces of Halibut Steak with Vegetables*
1 cup of Stovetop Spinach Casserole*
1 small baked potato
1 slice of whole-grain bread
1 piece of fruit
No-cal beverage

1800-Calorie Rotation

MENU **1**

Breakfast

8 ounces of skim or low-fat milk
1 poached egg
2 slices of whole-wheat toast
1 teaspoon of preserves
½ grapefruit
Coffee or tea

Lunch

6 ounces of Paprika Chicken*
1 cup of Potato Salad*
1 cup of cooked asparagus
1 cup of tossed salad
Lo-Cal Salad Dressing
1 pear
No-cal beverage

Dinner

1 cup of Egg Drop Soup*
1½ cups of Oriental Stir-Fry*
1 cup of Chinese Fried Rice*
½ cup of pineapple
3 Chewy Raisin Cookies*
8 ounces of skim or low-fat milk

MENU 2

Breakfast

8 ounces of skim or low-fat milk
1 cup of hot cereal
3 tablespoons of raisins
1 slice of whole-wheat toast
1 tablespoon of peanut butter
Coffee or tea

Lunch

4 ounces of Pepper Beef Burger*
1 whole-grain bun
1 cup of steamed cauliflower
Spinach Caesar Salad*
1 orange
Coffee or tea

Dinner

6 ounces of Broiled Snapper*
1 small baked potato
1 cup of tossed salad
Lo-Cal Salad Dressing
1 slice of whole-grain bread
1 apple
1 serving Honeydew De-Light*
No-cal beverage

MENU 3

Breakfast

8 ounces of skim or low-fat milk
1½ ounces of dry cereal
1 banana
1 slice of whole-wheat toast
1 teaspoon of preserves
Coffee or tea

Lunch

1 cup of soup (your choice)
4 ounces of roast turkey
2 slices of whole-grain bread
Lettuce, sprouts, and Dijon mustard
Unlimited free vegetables
1 pear
No-cal beverage

Dinner

5 ounces of Cantonese Chicken Stir-Fry*
1 cup of steamed carrots
1 slice of whole-grain bread or 1 whole-grain roll
2 Apple-Nut Bran Squares*

8 ounces of skim or low-fat milk
No-cal beverage

MENU **4**

Breakfast

1 German Fruit Puff*
8 ounces of skim or low-fat milk
Coffee or tea

Lunch

5 ounces of Savory Turkey Roll*
1 cup of broccoli
1 slice of whole-wheat bread
½ cup of brown rice
1 apple
No-cal beverage

Dinner

4 ounces of Veal in Mushroom Sauce*
1 cup of new potatoes and peas
1 cup of cooked cabbage
½ cup of Green Beans Almondine*
½ cup of sliced apricots
8 ounces of skim or low-fat milk
No-cal beverage

MENU **5**

Breakfast

8 ounces of skim or low-fat milk
1 cup of berries
1 bagel
2 tablespoons of cream cheese
Coffee or tea

Lunch

1 cup of Broccoli-Cauliflower Soup*
1 cup of carrots
4 ounces of baked fish
1 slice of whole-grain bread
1 orange
No-cal beverage

Dinner

4 ounces of Slim Southern-Style Fried Chicken*
1 cup of brown rice
1 cup of cooked asparagus
1 cup of tossed salad
Lo-Cal Salad Dressing
2 canned pear halves
No-cal beverage

MENU **6**

Breakfast

2 Whole-Wheat Breakfast Cakes*
2 tablespoons of maple syrup
8 ounces of skim or low-fat milk
½ grapefruit
Coffee or tea

Lunch

1 cup of soup (your choice)
2 turkey and sprout sandwiches, open-faced: each
with 1 slice of whole-grain bread, 1 ounce of turkey,
and Dijon mustard
1 cup of brussels sprouts

½ cup of pineapple
1 serving of Honeydew De-Light*
No-cal beverage

Dinner

4 ounces of Sesame Scallops*
1 baked potato
Spinach Caesar Salad*
Choice of assorted vegetable relishes: carrots, celery,
radishes, cucumber, etc.
1 slice of Pineapple Bread*
No-cal beverage

RECIPES

Soups

BROCCOLI-CAULIFLOWER SOUP

¾ pound of fresh chopped
broccoli
¾ pound of fresh chopped
cauliflower
⅓ cup of chopped onion
1½ cups of bouillon
¼ teaspoon of ground mace

3 cups of skim milk
1 tablespoon of cornstarch
½ teaspoon of salt
⅛ teaspoon of pepper
⅓ cup of shredded Swiss
cheese

Cook broccoli, cauliflower, and onion in the bouillon until
tender. Pour half the vegetables, along with half the bouillon,
into a blender or food processor and blend until smooth. Remove, and blend the remaining vegetable mixture, along with the
mace. Return all of blended mixture to pan.

Blend ½ cup of milk with cornstarch and add to vegetables.
Add remaining milk, salt, and pepper, and cook until thick and
hot, stirring occasionally. Blend in cheese and stir until melted.

Makes 8 servings at 71 calories per serving.

EGG DROP SOUP

1¼ cups of bouillon   2 tablespoons of chopped
1¼ cups of water   green onion
                                1 egg, slightly beaten

Combine bouillon and water in saucepan and bring to boil. Add
green onion, and reduce heat. Gently stir in beaten egg, and
simmer for three minutes or until egg is set. Serve immediately.
Makes 4 servings at 35 calories per serving.

MUSHROOM CLAM CHOWDER

½ cup of fresh mushrooms,   ⅛ teaspoon of pepper
    chopped   ⅛ teaspoon of cayenne
1 teaspoon of vegetable oil   1⅓ cups of nonfat dry milk
7-ounce can of minced   powder
    clams   1½ cups of cold water
½ cup of celery, chopped   1 tablespoon of cornstarch
⅓ cup of onion, chopped   2 tablespoons of minced
¼ teaspoon of salt   fresh parsley

Heat oil in saucepan and sauté mushrooms. Stir in undrained
clams, celery, onion, salt, pepper, and cayenne. Cover and let
simmer for 5 minutes. Mix together milk powder, water, and
cornstarch. (You may substitute 1½ cups of skim milk for the
milk powder and water.) Stir milk mixture into saucepan and
simmer over low heat until soup thickens. Pour into serving
bowls and top each serving with ½ tablespoon of minced parsley.
Makes 4 servings at 142 calories per serving.

Salads

CHICKEN AND SWISS SALAD

½ cup of plain yogurt
2 tablespoons of mayonnaise
1 tablespoon of fresh chopped parsley
1 teaspoon of horseradish
1 teaspoon of prepared mustard
¼ teaspoon of rosemary
¼ teaspoon of garlic powder

1 head of lettuce
12 sliced green pepper rings
6 slices of Swiss cheese, 1 ounce each
6 slices of sweet red onion
6 slices of cooked chicken or turkey, 1 ounce each
24 sliced cucumber rounds, ¼ inch thick
12 tomato slices

Blend together yogurt, mayonnaise, parsley, horseradish, mustard, rosemary, and garlic. Cover and chill while preparing the rest of the salad.

Remove core of lettuce head. Cut lettuce crosswise to get 6 slices, ½ inch thick. Place lettuce slices on serving plates. Top each lettuce slice with 2 green pepper rings, 1 slice of cheese, 1 slice of onion, 1 slice of chicken or turkey, 4 slices of cucumber, and 2 slices of tomato. Top each serving with 2 tablespoons of yogurt mixture.

Makes 6 servings at 224 calories per serving.

POTATO SALAD

3 medium-sized cooked potatoes, diced
¼ cup of chopped green onion
⅔ cup of chopped celery
1 tablespoon of mayonnaise

1 teaspoon of prepared mustard
1 teaspoon of dillweed
½ teaspoon of garlic powder

Combine all ingredients in a large bowl, and chill at least one hour.

Makes 4 servings, 1 cup each, at 102 calories per serving.

SEASONED TOMATO SALAD

1 cup of fresh chopped
   tomato
½ teaspoon of basil
½ teaspoon of oregano

1½ teaspoons of lemon juice
Several sprigs of fresh
   parsley, chopped

Combine all ingredients, cover, and let marinate in the refrigerator for an hour or more.

   Makes 1 serving of 52 calories.

SPINACH CAESAR SALAD

1 clove of garlic
10 ounces of fresh spinach
4 tablespoons of chopped
   onion
3 tablespoons of
   mayonnaise
¼ cup of Italian salad
   dressing

1 tablespoon of lemon or
   lime juice
¼ teaspoon of salt
⅛ teaspoon of black pepper
3 slices of whole-wheat
   bread, toasted, cubed
3 tablespoons of grated
   Parmesan cheese

Cut garlic clove in half and rub salad bowl with the cut ends. Discard garlic. Trim and shred spinach, and add to salad bowl. Add onion. Combine mayonnaise, salad dressing, lemon or lime juice, salt, and pepper, and pour over spinach. Toss warm toasted bread cubes with cheese, and pour onto salad.

   Makes 8 sevings at 67 calories per serving.

Main Courses

BAKED FISH IN SPRING HERBS

1 pound of fish fillets (sole
   or flounder works best)
1 tablespoon of vegetable
   oil or butter

1 lemon
1 teaspoon each of dried
   parsley, chives, and
   rosemary

Melt butter and pour into shallow baking dish. Arrange fish in dish. Cut lemon in half, and squeeze over the fish about 1 tablespoon of juice from one-half of the lemon. Sprinkle with herbs. Slice the remaining lemon into thin slices, and arrange on top of the fish.

Bake at 500 degrees for 12 to 15 minutes, or until fish flakes easily with fork.

Makes 4 servings of 4 ounces each, at about 115 calories per serving.

BROILED SNAPPER

2 pounds of snapper fillets	1¼ teaspoons of paprika
⅔ cup of tomato juice	⅛ teaspoon of salt
3 tablespoons of vinegar	⅛ teaspoon of black pepper

Cut fillets into 8 pieces. Arrange in shallow baking dish. Combine remaining ingredients and pour over fish. Marinate covered in refrigerator for 1 hour, turning once. Remove fish and place on broiler pan. Brush with marinade and broil 4 to 5 minutes, about 4 inches from heat. Turn and baste again with marinade. Broil another 4 to 5 minutes, or until fish flakes easily with a fork.

Makes 8 servings at 104 calories per serving.

CHEDDAR CHILI PIE

1 pound of lean ground beef or veal	2 tablespoons of chili powder
1 large onion, or 4 green onions, chopped	1 teaspoon of cumin
2 cloves of garlic, chopped fine	¼ teaspoon of cayenne
1 can (28 ounces) of tomatoes	½ teaspoon of crushed red pepper
1 can (15 ounces) of kidney beans, with juice	½ teaspoon of black pepper
1¼ cups of cornmeal	Dash Tabasco™ sauce
1 cup of grated cheddar cheese	1¼ cups of skim milk
	2 eggs, lightly beaten
	Salt and pepper to taste

Sauté beef, onion, and garlic until brown. Drain off fat. Add tomatoes, beans and bean juice, ¾ cup of cornmeal, ½ cup of cheese, and spices. Cook over low heat, stirring occasionally, for about 15 minutes. Pour into casserole dish.

In the same saucepan, combine the milk, the rest of the cornmeal, and salt and pepper to taste. Stir over low heat until the mixture thickens a little. Add the remaining cheese and the eggs, stirring until smooth. Pour this over the ground-beef mixture. Bake uncovered at 375 degrees for 30 minutes or until crust is lightly browned.

Makes 8 servings at 308 calories per serving.

CHICKEN CORDON BLEU

4 chicken breasts, skinned and boned	½ teaspoon of garlic powder
Nonstick vegetable cooking spray	½ teaspoon of onion powder
4 thin slices of ham, ½ ounce each	¼ teaspoon each of salt and black pepper
4 thin slices of Swiss cheese, ½ ounce each	1 egg
⅔ cup of whole-wheat flour	2 teaspoons of water
	⅔ cup of dry bread crumbs, sifted

Pound chicken breasts with mallet and cut each breast in half. Spray skillet with cooking spray, and lightly brown chicken on both sides. Remove from pan.

Place a slice of ham on each of four pieces of chicken; place a slice of cheese on top of each piece of ham. Top each with one of the remaining chicken halves, and pat dry.

Combine flour and seasonings in a shallow bowl. In another bowl, lightly beat egg and water together with 10 or 11 strokes. Place the bread crumbs, finely sifted, in a third bowl. Dip the chicken into the flour, carefully coating all sides and then removing excess flour. Slide chicken through egg mixture, and let excess drip off. Then dip in bread crumbs. Place on oven-proof platter and let stand for 15 minutes. Preheat oven to 350 degrees and bake chicken for 15 minutes.

Serves 4 at 316 calories per serving.

CHICKEN DIVAN

1¼ pounds of fresh broccoli
1½ cups of cold water
3 tablespoons of cornstarch
⅔ cup of skim milk
⅛ teaspoon of nutmeg
⅛ teaspoon of pepper
12 ounces of thinly sliced cooked chicken, white meat only (1 pound raw)

2 tablespoons of dry sherry
1½ teaspoons (1½ cubes) of instant chicken bouillon granules
¼ cup of grated Parmesan cheese

Cut broccoli into flowerets. Put 1½ cups of cold water in the bottom of a steamer, and heat to boiling. Steam broccoli until just tender. Drain and save the juice. Arrange broccoli in an 8-inch-square baking dish.

In a saucepan, heat the broccoli juice, adding, if necessary, enough additional cold water to make 1⅓ cups of juice. Stir in cornstarch. Add milk, sherry, bouillon granules, nutmeg, and pepper, stirring until thickened. Pour half the sauce over the broccoli. Layer chicken slices on top, then pour on remaining sauce. Sprinkle with cheese and paprika.

Bake, uncovered, at 350 degrees for 20 minutes.

Makes 6 servings at 166 calories per serving.

CHICKEN OAHU

4 boneless, skinned chicken breasts
1 can (8 ounces) of unsweetened pineapple chunks, undrained
½ cup of onions, sliced thin

1 sweet red pepper, chopped
¼ cup of lemon juice
¼ cup of orange juice

Combine all ingredients in a large casserole. Marinate, covered and refrigerated, for 2 hours, stirring occasionally. Place casse-

role in 325-degree oven for 1 hour, or until chicken is tender.
Makes 4 servings at 161 calories per serving.

CHICKEN PAPRIKA

1 teaspoon of butter	⅛ teaspoon of rosemary,
12 ounces of cooked	crushed
chicken pieces, white	Dash of salt
meat only (1 pound raw)	Dash of black pepper
1 teaspoon of paprika	Garlic powder to taste

Melt butter in small saucepan. Toss in chicken, coating with
butter. Stir in seasonings. Serve warm or cold.

Makes 2 to 4 servings; 3 ounces will contain 138 calories,
and 6 ounces will contain 276 calories.

CHICKEN SESAME

3 pounds of chicken pieces, skinned	¼ teaspoon each of onion powder, thyme, marjoram, and salt
½ cup of bread crumbs or Pepperidge Farm stuffing mix	½ teaspoon of dried parsley
⅛ cup of ground sesame seeds	½ teaspoon of dry mustard
	⅛ teaspoon of black pepper
1 clove of garlic, chopped fine	1 small egg, lightly beaten

Combine dry ingredients and seasonings; mix well. Place a layer
of chicken pieces in the bottom of a large casserole dish. Brush
the chicken with the beaten egg. Sprinkle with some of the
sesame mixture. Continue layering chicken, egg, and sesame
mixture until all ingredients are used up.

Bake covered at 300 degrees for 1½ to 2 hours, or until
chicken is tender.

Makes 8 servings at approximately 210 calories per serving.

CHICKEN TERIYAKI

4 chicken breasts, skinned
1 tablespoon of vegetable oil
2 tablespoons of soy sauce
1 large clove of garlic, crushed
1 tablespoon of fresh ginger, grated

Combine all ingredients except the chicken in a large bowl, and mix well. Add the chicken and marinate at least 4 hours in the refrigerator, stirring occasionally. Line a baking pan with foil and arrange chicken pieces on it. Baste each piece with the marinade. Bake at 350 degrees for 45 minutes, or until chicken is tender, basting frequently with the marinade.

Makes 4 servings at 154 calories per serving.

HALIBUT STEAK WITH VEGETABLES

2 pounds of halibut steaks
Nonstick vegetable cooking spray
⅔ cup of onion, sliced thin
1½ cups of fresh mushrooms, chopped
⅓ cup of tomato, chopped
⅓ cup of green pepper, chopped
¼ cup of fresh parsley, chopped
3 tablespoons of pimiento, chopped
⅓ cup of dry white wine
2 tablespoons of lemon or lime juice
1 teaspoon of salt
¼ teaspoon of dillweed
⅛ teaspoon of pepper
Lemon or lime wedges

Cut steaks into 8 pieces. Spray baking dish with cooking spray. Line bottom of dish with onion. Place fish on top of onion. Combine tomato, green pepper, parsley, and pimiento, and spread over fish. Blend wine, lemon or lime juice, and seasonings, and pour over vegetables. Bake at 350 degrees for 25 minutes, or until fish flakes easily with a fork. Serve with lemon or lime wedges.

Makes 8 servings at 137 calories per serving.

LEAN AND PERFECT PIZZA

Topping

½ pound of extra-lean
    ground beef
1 clove of garlic, minced
⅓ cup of chopped onion
1 can (16 ounces) of
    tomatoes, chopped
⅓ cup of chopped green
    pepper

1¼ teaspoons of oregano
1 teaspoon of basil
½ teaspoon of fennel seed
⅛ teaspoon of salt
1 cup shredded mozzarella
    cheese (4 ounces)

Crust

1 cup of whole-wheat
    flour
½ package of dry yeast
Dash salt
⅓ cup of warm water

1½ teaspoons of vegetable
    oil
Nonstick vegetable cooking
    spray

Brown beef, garlic, and onion in saucepan. Drain well. Stir in undrained tomatoes, green pepper, oregano, basil, fennel, and the salt. Bring to a boil. Then reduce heat and simmer gently, uncovered, for 30 minutes.

Meanwhile, combine ⅞ cup of the flour with the yeast and the salt. Add the warm water and oil. Beat at low speed with an electric mixer for 30 seconds, then beat at high speed for 3 minutes. Add as much of the remaining flour as you can stir in with a spoon. Turn out onto a floured board and knead in enough flour to make smooth, elastic dough (about 6 minutes). Cover dough and let stand in a warm place for 10 minutes. Roll dough into a 13-inch circle. Transfer to a pizza pan or a baking sheet sprayed with cooking spray. Turn up edges of the crust slightly. Bake at 425 degrees for 12 minutes, or until lightly browned.

Pour meat mixture onto crust, top with cheese, and bake for 15 more minutes, or until bubbly. Slice and serve.

Makes 4 servings at 354 calories per serving.

MEDLEY CASSEROLE

2 medium potatoes, cubed (leave skins on!)	½ teaspoon of rosemary
1 medium carrot, sliced in ¼-inch rounds	¼ teaspoon of salt
	¼ teaspoon of black pepper
1 stalk of celery, chopped	1 pound of fish fillets
1 onion, sliced in ¼-inch rounds	1 medium green pepper, chopped fine
1½ tablespoons of butter	1 tablespoon of lemon juice
1 teaspoon of dillweed	
1 teaspoon of basil	1 medium tomato, chopped fine

Layer potatoes, carrot, celery, and onion in an 8-inch-square baking dish. Melt butter and combine with dill, basil, rosemary, salt, and pepper. Spoon half of the seasoned butter over the vegetables. Cover and bake at 425 degrees for 25 minutes.

Arrange fish fillets on top of the vegetables and sprinkle with lemon juice. Spoon the remaining seasoned butter over the fish. Top with chopped green pepper. Cover and bake for 15 more minutes or until fish flakes easily with a fork. Uncover and add chopped tomato. Bake 5 minutes more, or until tomato is hot and vegetables are tender.

Makes 4 servings at 201 calories per serving.

ORIENTAL STIR-FRY

¾ pound of top round steak	2 tablespoons of soy sauce
½ cup of water	2 tablespoons of dry sherry
2 cups of broccoli flowerets	2 tablespoons of cooking oil
2 medium carrots, sliced	
1 teaspoon of cornstarch	1 medium onion, cut into thin wedges
¼ teaspoon of sugar	

Slice beef across the grain into thin, bite-sized pieces. Set aside. Bring water to a boil, and steam broccoli and carrots over hot water for 3 minutes. In a small bowl or measuring cup, combine cornstarch, sugar, soy sauce, and sherry, and reserve.

Preheat a wok or skillet over high heat for 1 minute. Add 1 tablespoon of the oil. Add vegetables, including onion, and stir-fry for several minutes, until just tender. Remove vegetables. Add remaining oil to skillet. Add beef and brown, stirring constantly. Add soy mixture, still stirring constantly, and stir until sauce thickens. Return vegetables to wok or skillet, cover, and cook 1 minute more.

Makes 4 servings at 292 calories per serving.

PAPRIKA PORK GOULASH

1 pound of pork tenderloin	1 tablespoon of cornstarch
Nonstick vegetable cooking spray	1 cup of plain yogurt
	¼ cup of fresh parsley
1 large onion, chopped	2½ cups of cooked
¾ cup of bouillon	whole-wheat noodles
1 tablespoon of paprika	

Trim all visible fat from pork. Slice pork diagonally into ¼-inch slices. Spray skillet with cooking spray, and heat over medium heat. Brown meat in skillet, stirring occasionally. Remove meat from pan. Place onions in pan and cook lightly until clear. (You may add some of the bouillon if there isn't enough fat to cook the onions.)

Return meat to skillet. Add bouillon and paprika. Cover and let simmer 15 to 20 minutes, until pork is tender. Take 6 tablespoons of bouillon out of pan and reserve in small container in refrigerator.

Blend cornstarch into yogurt in a small bowl. Take the reserved bouillon out of the refrigerator and stir into the yogurt mixture, 1 tablespoon at a time. Add yogurt mixture to skillet and heat through. Stir in parsley, and serve over hot noodles.

Makes 5 servings at 296 calories per serving.

PEPPER BEEF BURGERS

¼ cup of fine dry bread crumbs
2 tablespoons of low-fat dry milk
½ teaspoon of basil
½ teaspoon of oregano
½ teaspoon of garlic powder
⅛ teaspoon of salt
⅛ teaspoon of black pepper
¾ pound of ground chuck or ground round
2 medium onions, sliced thin
¾ cup of tomato sauce
¼ cup of red wine
1 large green pepper, cut into julienne strips

Combine bread crumbs, milk, and seasonings in bowl. Add meat and mix well. Shape into four patties, ¾ inch thick. Brown patties on both sides in skillet. Drain off fat. Add onions to skillet. Blend together tomato sauce and wine, and pour into skillet. Cover and cook on low heat for about 10 minutes. Top with green pepper, cover, and cook 10 minutes more.

Makes 4 servings at 219 calories per serving.

QUICK SKILLET

2 cups of lean roasted pork, cut into 1-inch cubes
2 onions, cut into chunks
2 tablespoons of soy sauce
2 tablespoons of water
¼ cup of unsweetened pineapple juice
¾ pound of fresh asparagus, cut into 1-inch lengths
⅓ cup of fresh mushrooms, sliced
¾ cup of cubed tomato pieces
1 teaspoon of cornstarch
¼ cup of white wine or vinegar

Combine pork, onions, soy sauce, and water in skillet. Cook on high heat for 1 or 2 minutes. Add juice, asparagus, and mushrooms, and cook 6 minutes more. Add tomato. Dissolve cornstarch in wine and stir into meat mixture. Stirring constantly, cook for 2 or 3 minutes more, until sauce thickens, and vegetables are tender.

Makes 4 servings at 257 calories per serving.

ROLLED HAM AND VEGETABLES

¼ cup of chopped
   cucumber
¼ cup of chopped tomato
⅓ cup of sliced fresh
   mushrooms
2 tablespoons of sliced
   ripe olives
2 tablespoons of green
   onions, chopped

¼ cup of low-calorie Italian
   salad dressing
4 large lettuce leaves, from
   outer part of head
1 6-ounce package of sliced,
   cooked ham (8 slices)
1 cup of shredded mozzarella
   cheese

Combine cucumber, tomato, mushrooms, olives, green onion, and salad dressing in a bowl. Chill, covered, for at least 2 hours. (You can keep this overnight in the refrigerator, if you wish.)

Top a lettuce leaf with two slices of ham. Drain the vegetables, and place ¼ cup of the mixture in the center of the ham. Sprinkle ¼ cup of cheese on top. Roll up, while turning the edges of the lettuce inward to seal the ends. Secure with a toothpick.

Makes 4 servings of one roll each at 205 calories per serving.

SAVORY TURKEY ROLL

1¼ pounds of boned turkey
   breast
¼ teaspoon of garlic
   powder
⅛ teaspoon of black
   pepper
¼ cup of chopped onion
3 tablespoons of chopped
   fresh parsley

2 ounces of cheddar cheese
   (4 half-ounce slices)
1 cup of tomato juice
2 teaspoons of Worcestershire
   sauce
Dash of Tabasco™ sauce

Preheat oven to 350 degrees. Sprinkle turkey meat with garlic, pepper, onion, and parsley. Top with cheese slices. Roll up and place in small baking dish. Secure with toothpicks or skewers if necessary. Combine remaining ingredients and pour over turkey roll. Bake covered for 2 hours, basting occasionally. Uncover and bake another hour. Slice and serve.

Makes 4 servings at 209 calories per serving.

SEAFOOD ITALIA

Nonstick vegetable cooking spray
2 pounds of fish fillets
¼ cup of unsalted tomato juice
3 tablespoons of steak sauce

1½ tablespoons of Italian salad dressing
⅛ teaspoon of curry powder
Dash of hot pepper sauce

Spray nonstick broiler pan with cooking spray. Arrange fillets on pan. Combine remaining ingredients, and pour half of mixture over the fish. Broil 4 to 5 minutes, then turn fillets over, cover with the remaining sauce, and broil another 4 to 5 minutes, or until fish flakes easily with a fork.

Makes 8 servings of 4 ounces each, including sauce, at 109 calories per serving.

SESAME SCALLOPS

1 pound of large fresh scallops
3 tablespoons of sherry
2 tablespoons of cooking oil
1 tablespoon of sesame seeds, crushed
2 teaspoons of grated onion
1 clove of garlic, crushed

¼ teaspoon of salt
⅛ teaspoon of pepper
1 green pepper, cut into chunks
1 sweet red pepper, cut into chunks
1 can (8 ounces) of unsweetened pineapple chunks, drained
12 cherry tomatoes

Combine sherry, oil, sesame seeds, onion, garlic, salt, and pepper in large plastic bowl. Add scallops and pepper chunks, and marinate in refrigerator for 3 or 4 hours, stirring occasionally. Thread scallops, peppers, and pineapple on 6 skewers. Place skewers in baking pan and pour marinade in. Bake at 425 degrees for 10 minutes, or until scallops are tender, turning skewers occasionally. Place two tomatoes on the end of each skewer, and return to oven for 5 more minutes.

Makes 6 servings at about 174 calories per serving.

SHRIMP JAMBALAYA

½ cup of chopped green onion
¼ cup of chopped green pepper
1 clove of garlic, minced
2 tablespoons of butter
2 tablespoons of whole-wheat flour
1 can (16 ounces) of stewed tomatoes, undrained
1 cup cooked, cubed ham
½ cup of water

2 bay leaves
½ teaspoon of thyme
½ teaspoon of basil
¼ teaspoon of dillweed
¼ teaspoon of crushed red pepper
¼ teaspoon of salt
⅛ teaspoon of black pepper
Dash of Tabasco™ sauce
1 cup of uncooked brown rice, washed and drained
1 pound of shelled shrimp

Melt butter in saucepan and brown onion, green pepper, and garlic until tender. Blend in all remaining ingredients except the shrimp. Bring to a boil, then reduce heat and simmer for about 30 minutes, stirring frequently. Add shrimp and cook 15 minutes more, or until rice and shrimp are cooked.

Makes 6 servings at 283 calories per serving.

SLIM SOUTHERN-STYLE FRIED CHICKEN

4 pounds of chicken pieces, skinned

Water
½ cup of bread crumbs

¼ teaspoon of thyme
½ teaspoon of paprika
¼ teaspoon of salt

¼ teaspoon of marjoram
¼ teaspoon of celery seed
⅛ teaspoon of black pepper

Brush chicken pieces with water to moisten. Combine remaining ingredients in a large bowl. Dredge chicken in the coating, and arrange on a nonstick baking sheet. Bake at 375 degrees for 45 minutes, or until crisp on the outside and tender inside.

Makes 8 servings at about 186 calories per serving.

SPICY ORANGE PORK

6 pork chops, top loin, ½ inch thick
Nonstick vegetable spray
¼ teaspoon of salt
¼ teaspoon of pepper
¼ cup of unsweetened orange juice

2 medium oranges
1 cup of water
2 teaspoons of sugar
1 tablespoon of cornstarch
1 cup of unsweetened orange juice
¼ teaspoon of allspice

Trim pork chops of all visible fat. Spray skillet with nonstick vegetable spray, and heat over medium heat. Brown chops on both sides. Sprinkle with salt and pepper, and add ¼ cup of the orange juice. Cover and let simmer 25 minutes or until tender.

Meanwhile, remove a thin layer of peel from one orange, and slice the peel into julienne strips. Simmer strips in water for 15 minutes, drain, and set aside. Peel and section both oranges, and cut the sections into ½-inch chunks.

Combine sugar, cornstarch, and 1 cup of orange juice in another saucepan, stirring constantly over medium heat until thickened. Add the julienned orange peel, orange chunks, and allspice. Simmer 1 or 2 minutes longer, stirring occasionally. Remove chops to serving dish, and top with sauce.

Makes 6 servings at 205 calories per serving.

VEAL IN MUSHROOM SAUCE

¾ pound of boneless
   veal-leg round steak
2 teaspoons of butter
1½ teaspoons of
   Worcestershire sauce
1 clove of garlic,
   chopped fine
1 medium onion, sliced
   into rings
1 cup of sliced fresh
   mushrooms

⅓ cup of beef bouillon
1 tablespoon of lemon or
   lime juice
2 teaspoons of cornstarch
¼ cup of cold water
2 cups of cooked
   whole-wheat noodles
Lemon or lime wedges

Trim visible fat from veal, and cut into 4 pieces. Pound meat with a mallet to ¼-inch thickness.

Melt butter in skillet. Add Worcestershire sauce, garlic, and onion. Cook over medium heat until onion is clear. Add veal and brown on both sides. Pour mushrooms over veal, and add bouillon and lemon or lime juice. Reduce heat to low, cover, and simmer for about 5 minutes, until meat is cooked.

Combine cornstarch and water, and stir onto meat. Heat and stir until bubbly and thick. Serve over hot noodles, garnished with lemon or lime wedges.

Makes 4 servings at approximately 290 calories per serving.

VEAL STEW

1¼ pounds of lean boneless
   veal, cut into 1-inch
   cubes
2 small cloves of garlic,
   minced
½ medium onion,
   chopped
2 teaspoons of butter
1¾ cups of bouillon
3 tablespoons of white
   wine

2 medium potatoes,
   cubed
2 medium carrots, sliced
1 cup of frozen or fresh peas
1 cup of fresh mushrooms,
   halved
2 tablespoons of fresh parsley,
   chopped
1 teaspoon of marjoram
2 tablespoons of water
1 tablespoon of cornstarch

In a large kettle brown the meat, garlic, and onions in butter. Add bouillon and wine, and bring to a boil. Reduce heat, cover, and simmer for 30 minutes. Add remaining vegetables and seasonings. Cover and cook another 30 minutes, or until meat is cooked and vegetables are tender. Skim any visible fat off the top. Combine the 2 tablespoons of water and the cornstarch; add to the stew and stir until thickened.

Makes 6 servings at 311 calories per serving.

Vegetables

CARROTS ALOHA

1 cup of carrots
¼ cup of water
1 tablespoon of fresh orange juice
2 teaspoons of fresh lemon juice
2 lemon slices
4 orange slices

Cut carrots in quarters lengthwise, then cut into 1-inch strips. Bring water to a boil in saucepan. Place carrots in water, reduce heat, cover, and cook until just tender. Add juices and stir. Place sliced lemon and orange rounds on top of carrots, cover, and cook 2 or 3 minutes more.

Makes one serving of 52 calories.

CHINESE FRIED RICE

1 cup of brown rice
2 cups of water
Nonstick vegetable cooking spray
2 eggs, beaten
2 large onions, chopped
2 teaspoons of vegetable oil
¼ cup of water
¾ cup of celery, chopped
½ cup of green pepper, chopped
1 clove of garlic, minced
3 green onions, chopped

Bring 2 cups of water to a boil, add rice, and reduce heat. Let simmer for 40 to 45 minutes, until tender. Set aside.

Spray a large skillet with cooking spray. Add eggs and cook over low heat without stirring. When eggs are set, remove from skillet, crumble with a fork, and reserve. Brown onions in skillet with the oil. Add remaining ingredients, and heat to boiling. Add cooked rice. Reduce heat and simmer 1 minute. Stir in egg. Remove from heat, cover, and let stand 5 minutes.

Makes 8 servings at 92 calories per serving.

HERB AND GARLIC BRUSSELS SPROUTS

¾ pound of fresh or
  frozen brussels sprouts
1 small onion, sliced thin
1 clove of garlic, minced
2½ teaspoons of butter

¼ teaspoon of thyme
¼ teaspoon of oregano
⅛ teaspoon of salt
⅛ teaspoon of black pepper

Steam brussels sprouts and onions over boiling water for about 20 minutes, or until tender.

Melt butter in saucepan, add garlic, and sauté until browned. Add steamed vegetables and seasonings. Cook 4 minutes, or until vegetables are heated through, stirring occasionally.

Makes 4 servings at about 70 calories per serving.

ISLAND RICE

1 cup of brown rice
2 cups of bouillon
½ medium onion, sliced
  thin

1 tablespoon of toasted,
  shredded coconut

Wash rice, draining off excess liquid. Bring bouillon and onion to a boil in a saucepan. Add rice and reduce heat to low. Simmer for 40 to 50 minutes, or until rice is tender. Top with toasted coconut.

Makes 4 servings of ½ cup each, at 106 calories per serving.

OVEN-FRIED POTATOES

4 medium potatoes, skins on
1 tablespoon of oil
⅛ teaspoon of garlic powder
⅛ teaspoon of onion powder
1 to 1½ teaspoons of paprika (to taste)
Salt and pepper to taste

Slice potatoes lengthwise into eighths.

Line a shallow baking pan with foil, and put all ingredients into the pan, tossing well to coat the potatoes with the oil and seasonings.

Bake at 325 degrees for 1 hour, or at a higher temperature for less time if you wish. Adjust seasonings if necessary.

Makes 4 servings at 115 calories per serving.

PEAS AND PODS

1 package (10½ ounces) of frozen green peas
1 cup of fresh snow peas
1 small onion, sliced thin
1 teaspoon of basil

Cook frozen peas according to directions on package. At the same time, steam snow peas and onion over hot water until tender. When cooked, add snow peas and onion to frozen peas. Add basil, stir, and serve.

Makes 4 half-cup servings at approximately 54 calories per serving.

SPICY GREEN BEANS

¾ pound of fresh whole green beans	½ teaspoon of basil
¾ cup of unsalted tomato juice	¼ teaspoon of garlic powder
2 tablespoons of chopped onion	¼ teaspoon of salt
1 teaspoon of oregano	⅛ teaspoon of pepper
	1 tablespoon of grated Romano cheese

Wash and trim green beans and cut into 1-inch lengths. Combine beans and remaining ingredients in saucepan and bring to a boil. Reduce heat and simmer, covered, for 5 minutes. Uncover and continue to cook until beans are tender. Sprinkle with cheese.

Makes 3 servings at 47 calories per serving.

STOVETOP SPINACH CASSEROLE

¾ pound of fresh spinach	3 tablespoons of fresh onion, chopped fine
½ cup of bouillon	
2 tablespoons of mayonnaise	

Wash and trim spinach. Combine all ingredients in saucepan, and bring to a boil. Reduce heat immediately and simmer, uncovered, until most of the liquid has evaporated.

Makes 3 servings at 44 calories per serving.

Desserts

APPLE-NUT BRAN SQUARES

1 cup of 40% Bran Flakes
  or Raisin Bran
½ cup of wheat germ
½ cup of nonfat dry milk
  powder
½ cup of firmly packed
  brown sugar
½ cup of finely chopped
  apples, skins on
2 tablespoons of vegetable
  oil
1 tablespoon of dark
  molasses

½ teaspoon of baking
  powder
⅛ teaspoon of salt
2 beaten eggs
1¾ teaspoons of vanilla
⅓ cup of chopped pecans or
  walnuts
Nonstick vegetable cooking
  spray

Combine bran, wheat germ, milk, baking powder, and salt in a
large bowl. In a separate bowl, combine eggs, sugar, apples, oil,
molasses, and vanilla. Add egg mixture gradually to dry mixture, blending well. Add nuts. Spray a 9-inch-square baking pan
with cooking spray. Turn batter into pan and bake at 350 degrees
for 25 minutes. Cool and cut into 20 squares.

Makes 20 servings at approximately 85 calories per serving.

CHEWY RAISIN COOKIES

¼ cup of butter
⅓ cup of firmly packed
  brown sugar
1½ teaspoons of vanilla
1 egg
1¼ cups of whole-wheat
  flour

½ teaspoon of baking soda
¼ teaspoon of salt
½ teaspoon of cinnamon
½ cup of raisins

Preheat oven to 375 degrees. Beat together butter, sugar, vanilla,
and egg. Combine dry ingredients and add to butter mixture,

blending well. Stir in raisins. Drop by level teaspoonfuls onto nonstick, ungreased cookie sheets. Bake for 8 minutes, or until golden brown.

Makes 50 cookies at approximately 30 calories apiece.

HONEYDEW DE-LIGHT

1 medium honeydew or other melon (4 cups)
1 teaspoon of unflavored gelatin
2 tablespoons of water

2 tablespoons of lime or lemon juice
2 tablespoons of honey
Lime or lemon twists

Cut melon into cubes. Soften gelatin in water in glass dish. Place glass of gelatin in pan of water and heat until gelatin is dissolved, stirring constantly. Combine 1 cup of the melon cubes, lime or lemon juice, honey, and gelatin mixture in a blender, and blend on high for 30 seconds. Add remaining melon, and blend again until smooth. Pour into 8-inch-square pan, and place in freezer.

When mixture is almost firm, remove from pan and place in chilled bowl. Beat with electric mixer at high speed until smooth. Return to freezer pan, and freeze until firm (several hours). To serve, remove from freezer and let stand about 15 minutes at room temperature. Spoon into serving dishes. Garnish with lime or lemon twists.

Makes 6 servings at 61 calories per serving.

PINEAPPLE BREAD

2½ cups of whole-wheat flour
½ cup of 40% Bran Flakes or Raisin Bran
2 tablespoons of wheat germ

1 teaspoon of baking soda
1 teaspoon of baking powder
Pinch of salt
1 beaten egg

2 cartons (8 ounces each)
of pineapple yogurt
¼ cup of skim milk
2 tablespoons of vegetable
oil
2 tablespoons of molasses
2 tablespoons of honey

1 teaspoon of lime or lemon
juice
1 cup of raisins
½ cup of chopped pecans
½ cup of dates, chopped
Nonstick vegetable cooking
spray

Combine flour, bran, wheat germ, baking soda, baking powder, and salt in a large bowl. In another bowl, combine egg, yogurt, milk, oil, molasses, honey, and lime or lemon juice. Stir into dry ingredients. Add raisins, nuts, and dates. Spray 2 loaf pans with cooking spray, and turn batter into pans. Bake at 325 degrees for 1 hour, or until toothpick inserted in center comes out clean. Cool for 15 minutes, and remove from pans. Allow to cool completely on wire rack. Store overnight, wrapped well, before slicing.

Makes 30 servings at about 92 calories per serving.

TROPICAL COCONUT CRUST PIE

1 tablespoon of butter
1¼ cups of flaked coconut
1 can (20 ounces) of
crushed unsweetened
pineapple

Water
1 envelope of unflavored
gelatin
2 cartons (8 ounces each) of
orange yogurt

Preheat oven to 325 degrees. Melt butter and toss with coconut in a 9-inch pie plate. Press onto the bottom and the sides of the plate. Bake for 15 minutes, or until golden. Cool on wire rack.

Meanwhile, drain pineapple, and reserve juice. Add water to juice, if necessary, to make ¾ cup of liquid. Soften gelatin in liquid in a small saucepan. Cook over low heat until gelatin is dissolved, stirring constantly. Remove from heat and chill until partially set, to the consistency of unbeaten egg whites, then beat gelatin until fluffy. Fold in yogurt and pineapple, and pour into cooled crust. Chill until firm.

Makes 8 servings at 139 calories per serving.

Crackers and Pancakes

GERMAN FRUIT PUFF

½ cup of all-purpose flour
½ cup of whole-wheat flour
½ teaspoon of baking powder
½ teaspoon of salt

1 cup of skim milk
5 eggs
2 teaspoons of vegetable oil
3¼ cups of any variety of fresh fruit, sliced

Preheat oven to 425 degrees. Sift together flours, baking powder, and salt in mixing bowl. Stir in milk. Beat eggs in, one at a time. Heat oil over medium heat in a large, metal-handled skillet. Pour in batter and let cook 1 minute. Place skillet in oven and bake, uncovered, for 20 minutes, or until puff is golden brown. Top with fruit, and slice into 6 wedges.

Makes 6 servings at 207 calories per serving.

TOASTED OAT THINS

½ cup of quick-cooking rolled oats
⅓ cup of all-purpose unbleached, enriched flour
⅓ cup of whole-wheat flour
⅓ cup of wheat germ

1 tablespoon of sugar
1 tablespoon of sesame seeds, crushed
½ teaspoon of garlic powder
⅛ teaspoon of salt
¼ cup of butter
½ cup of cold water

Blend oats in a blender or food processor until evenly ground. Pour oats into mixing bowl. Add flours, wheat germ, sugar, sesame seed, garlic, and salt. Cut in butter until mixture has consistency of coarse bread crumbs. Gradually mix in cold water to form a dough. Shape the dough into a 9-inch-long roll. Wrap in plastic wrap and chill for at least 3 hours. Slice into ⅛-inch-thick rounds and place on foil-lined, ungreased baking sheet. Flatten with tines of a fork until thin. Bake at 375 degrees for 12 minutes, or until edges are nicely browned. Cool on wire rack.

Makes 6 dozen crackers at 19 calories each.

WHOLE-WHEAT BREAKFAST CAKES

1¼ cups of whole-wheat flour
2¼ teaspoons of baking powder
¼ teaspoon of salt

1 egg
1¼ cups of skim milk
Nonstick vegetable cooking spray

Combine flour, baking powder, and salt in mixing bowl. Beat together egg and milk, and stir into flour mixture to form lumpy batter. Spray nonstick skillet with cooking spray and heat over medium heat. Drop batter by spoonfuls onto skillet to make 4-inch pancakes. Reduce heat to low and cook until bubbles begin to form on cakes. Turn and cook on the other side until golden brown.

This makes 8 servings of cake at about 87 calories each.

13

Epilogue

Do you remember those five little words—my magical cure for obesity?

EAT LESS FAT AND WALK

Use the Rotation Diet periodically if you have more weight to lose than you can take off in twenty-one days. Then practice the magical cure on a daily basis, forever after. Of course, if walking is not your thing, do whatever you like in the way of brisk physical activity. But always pay attention to my words about fat in your diet. *You can't get fat if you don't eat fat!*

And remember that I'd like to hear from you when you finish the Rotation Diet (see Appendix B). Write to me, telling me how the Rotation Diet worked for you and join our follow-up study. Joining might help you stay at desirable weight and it will help us in our research on the effectiveness of the Rotation Diet.

Here's to your success! And I'm looking forward to hearing from you.

Appendix A

The Rotation Diet Quick Calorie Counter

Calorie Chart

FOOD	CALORIES
Apple, medium size with skin	80
Apple juice, canned, ½ cup	59
Applesauce, unsweetened, ½ cup	50
Apricots, dried, 4 large halves	59
Apricots, raw, without pits (3)	55
Artichoke, fresh, boiled	40
Artichoke hearts, frozen or water packed, 3 ounces (5)	20
Asparagus, fresh or frozen, 3 stalks	9
Avocado, ½ medium	185
Bacon, 1 thin slice cooked crisp and dry	30
Bagel, 3-inch diameter, egg or water	165
Baking powder, 1 teaspoon	5
Bamboo shoots, ½ pound	20
Banana, ½ small	41
Barbecue sauce, 1 cup	230
Barley, 1 cup uncooked	700
Bean sprouts, ½ cup	19
Beans, baby lima, 2 ounces	70
Beans, black-eyed peas, dry, cooked, 1 cup	190
Beans, navy, dry, cooked, 1 cup	225
Beans, red kidney, canned, 1 cup	230

Calorie Chart (Continued)

FOOD	CALORIES
Beef, lean, 3 ounces	165
Beef broth (bouillon), 8 ounces	23
Beets, ½ cup	27
Biscuits, 2-inch diameter, homemade	105
Biscuits, 2-inch diameter, from mix	90
Blackberries, fresh, 1 cup	85
Blueberries, fresh, ½ cup	45
Bran cereal, pure, ½ cup	95
Bread crumbs, dry, 1 cup	390
Bread, white, 1 slice	65
Bread, whole wheat, 1 slice	65
Broccoli, cooked, ½ cup	30
Brussels sprouts, ½ cup	28
Butter, 1 tablespoon	102
Buttermilk, skim, 1 cup	88
Cabbage, ½ cup	11
Cabbage, Chinese, ½ cup	6
Canadian bacon, 1 ounce	52
Cantaloupe, ½ medium	60
Carrots, ½ cup	23
Casaba melon, ⅛	38
Catsup, 1 tablespoon	16
Cauliflower, ½ cup	13
Caviar, 1 ounce	75
Celery, ½ cup	9
Cheese, blue, 1 ounce	100
Cheese, cheddar, 1-inch cube	68
Cheese, Gruyère, 1 ounce	115
Cheese, mozzarella, part skim, 1 ounce	80
Cheese, Parmesan, grated, 1 tablespoon	23
Cheese, provolone, 1 ounce	100
Cheese, ricotta, part skim, 1 cup	340
Cheese, Romano, 1 ounce	110
Cheese, Roquefort, 1 ounce	111
Cheese, Swiss, 1 ounce	104
CheezWhiz, 1 ounce	91
Cherries, fresh, ½ cup	41
Chicken, cooked, 1 ounce of meat, no skin	43
Chili sauce, 1 tablespoon	16
Chutney, 1 tablespoon	53
Clams, 4 or 5 medium	56
Clam juice, 1 cup	46
Cocoa, dry, 1 tablespoon	14
Cod, fresh, 4 ounces cooked	89

Calorie Chart *(Continued)*

FOOD	CALORIES
Coffee, 1 cup	2
Coffee, decaffeinated, 1 cup	3
Collard greens, cooked, 1 cup	58
Cottage cheese, low fat, 4 ounces	90
Cream substitute (Coffee-Mate), 1 teaspoon	11
Corn kernels, ½ cup	69
Corn on the cob, 1 medium	74
Corned beef, 2 ounces	200
Cornmeal, bolted, dry, 1 cup	440
Cornstarch, 1 tablespoon	30
Crabmeat, Alaskan, 4 ounces cooked	116
Crabmeat, lump, ½ cup cooked	50
Crackers, club, 1 piece	15
Crackers, graham, 1 piece	17
Crackers, saltines, 1 piece	12
Crackers, Melba Toast, 1 slice	15
Crackers, oyster, ½ cup	60
Crackers, Ritz, 1 piece	15
Crackers, whole wheat, 1 piece	16
Cranberries, ½ cup	22
Cranberry juice, ½ cup	82
Cream, half-and-half, 1 tablespoon	20
Cream, whipping, 1 tablespoon	45
Cream, sour, 1 tablespoon	29
Cream cheese, 1 ounce	106
Cucumber, ½ cup	8
Curry powder, 1 tablespoon	12
Dandelion greens, cooked, drained, 1 cup	35
Egg, 1 medium	72
Egg white, 1 medium	15
Egg yolk, 1 medium	52
Eggplant, 1 medium	92
Enchilada, 1 average	185
Endive, raw, 1 cup	10
English muffin	140
Farmer cheese, 1 tablespoon	19
Fat, vegetable, 1 tablespoon	111
Figs, fresh, 1 small	30
Flounder, 5 ounces cooked	118
Flour, buckwheat, light, sifted, 1 cup	340
Flour, carob, 1 ounce (1 cup = 5 ounces dry weight)	50
Flour, gluten, 1 ounce (1 cup = 5 ounces dry weight)	108
Flour, soybean, 1 ounce (1 cup defatted = 5 ounces dry weight)	90
Flour, wheat, 1 ounce (1 cup = 4 ounces dry weight)	102

Calorie Chart (Continued)

FOOD	CALORIES
Flour, self-rising, 1 ounce (1 cup = 4 ounces dry weight)	99
Frankfurter, 1, all beef, 1.5 ounces	142
Garlic, 1 ounce	39
Gelatin, 1 tablespoon	23
Ginger root, skinned, 1 ounce	14
Grapes, ½ cup (10)	34
Grape juice, sweetened, ½ cup	104
Grape juice, unsweetened, 4 ounces	80
Grapefruit, ½	55
Grapefruit sections, 1 cup	80
Green beans, ½ cup	18
Halibut, 4 ounces cooked	114
Ham, 2 ounces	106
Honey, 1 tablespoon	64
Honeydew melon, ⅛	50
Ice cream, rich, ½ cup	164
Ice milk, hardened, ½ cup	100
Jerusalem artichoke, ½ cup	25
Kale, cooked, 1 cup	45
Lamb, lean, cooked, 2 ounces	105
Leeks, sliced, 2 ounces	30
Lemon, 1 medium	20
Lemon juice, 1 tablespoon	4
Lettuce, soft, 1 head	23
Lettuce, iceberg, 8 ounces	30
Lettuce, iceberg, chopped, 1 cup	10
Lettuce, romaine, chopped, 1 cup	8
Lime, 1	19
Liver, calf, raw, 2 ounces	80
Liver, chicken, raw, 2 ounces	73
Lobster, 2 ounces cooked	52
Macaroni, cooked, ½ cup	78
Mandarin oranges, canned, low calorie, ½ cup	31
Mango, ½ cup	56
Maple syrup, 1 tablespoon	50
Margarine, 1 tablespoon	102
Margarine, imitation, 1 tablespoon	50
Margarine, whipped, 1 tablespoon	68
Mayonnaise, 1 tablespoon	101
Milk, goat, 1 cup	163
Milk, skim, 1 cup	80
Milk, 2% fat, 1 cup	120
Milk, whole, 1 cup	160

Calorie Chart *(Continued)*

FOOD	CALORIES
Mushrooms, canned, sliced, ½ cup	17
Mushrooms, fresh, sliced, ½ cup	13
Mustard greens, cooked, 1 cup	30
Nectarine, ½ cup	70
Nuts, almonds, chopped, 1 cup	775
Nuts, Brazil, 6–8 large	185
Nuts, cashews, roasted in oil, 1 cup	785
Nuts, coconut, shredded, not pressed down, 1 cup	275
Nuts, hazelnuts, chopped, 1 cup	730
Nuts, peanuts, raw, shelled, 1 ounce	155
Nuts, peanuts, roasted in oil, 1 cup	840
Nuts, peanuts, dry roasted, 1 ounce	170
Nuts, macadamia, 1 ounce	218
Nuts, pecans, shelled, halves, ½ cup	370
Nuts, pistachio, 1 tablespoon	46
Nuts, walnuts, chopped, 1 cup	785
Oil, vegetable, 1 tablespoon	120
Okra, 8 medium	24
Olives, 1 large	10
Onion, ½ cup	22
Onions, green, 3 small	14
Orange, 1	71
Orange juice, ½ cup	41
Orange sections, ½ cup	42
Oysters, raw, 1 medium	7
Pancakes, buckwheat, 1	55
Pancakes, plain, 1	60
Papaya, ½	60
Parsley, 1 tablespoon	1
Parsnip, ½ cup	51
Pea pods, ½ cup	50
Peach, fresh, 1 average	38
Peanut butter, 1 tablespoon	94
Pear, 1 fresh, 6 ounces	80
Pear, canned, water-packed, ½ cup	40
Peas, cooked, ½ cup	57
Pepper, green, 1 medium	16
Pepper, red, 1 medium	23
Persimmon, ½ cup	144
Pickles, dill, 1	3
Pie crust, 9-inch, 1	675
Pie crust, ⅙	112
Pimiento, ½ cup	31

Calorie Chart *(Continued)*

FOOD	CALORIES
Pineapple, ½ cup diced, fresh (about 1 slice, ¾ inch thick)	41
Pineapple, ½ cup, canned, water-packed	39
Plum, damson, 1 raw	33
Pompano, 4 ounces cooked	188
Popcorn, oil and salt, 1 cup	64
Popover, 1 average	112
Pork, roasted, 4 ounces	277
Pork, shoulder, lean, 4 ounces cooked	220
Pork sausage, 1 ounce	142
Potato, 1 medium	88
Potato chips, 10	113
Pound cake, 1 slice	150
Pretzels, 1 small	4
Prunes, cooked without sugar, 5 medium	119
Prune juice, ½ cup	88
Pumpkin, canned, ½ cup	40
Pumpkin and squash seeds, dry, hulled, 1 cup	775
Radish, 4 small	6
Raisins, 1 tablespoon	26
Raspberries, fresh, ½ cup	35
Raspberries, frozen, ½ cup	122
Rice, brown, ½ cup cooked	89
Rice, white, ½ cup cooked	82
Rice, blend of long grain and wild, ½ cup cooked	111
Rutabaga, diced, ½ cup	30
Salami, 1 slice (1 ounce)	90
Salmon, 2 ounces cooked	104
Salmon, smoked, 1 ounce	50
Salsify, canned, ½ cup	79
Salt, any quantity	0
Sardines, in oil, a 3¾-ounce can (6–8 sardines)	167
Sauerkraut, ½ cup	21
Scallops, raw, ½ cup	92
Sesame seeds, 1 ounce (2 tablespoons)	165
Shad, 4 ounces, baked	201
Shallots, 1 ounce	14
Shrimp, meat only, ½ cup, about 3½ ounces	91
Soft drinks, colas, 12 ounces	145
Soft drinks, ginger ale, 12 ounces	115
Soft drinks, root beer, 12 ounces	150
Sole, 4 ounces cooked	90
Spinach, trimmed, raw, 1 cup	14
Squab, meat only, 4 ounces cooked	161
Squash, acorn, ½ cup	56

Calorie Chart *(Continued)*

FOOD	CALORIES
Squash, yellow, ½ cup sliced	18
Squash, zucchini, ½ cup sliced thin	9
Sugar, brown, 1 tablespoon	49
Sugar, confectioners', 1 tablespoon	31
Sugar, granulated, 1 tablespoon	46
Sunflower seeds, dry, hulled, 1 cup	810
Sweetbreads, calf, 4 ounces cooked	188
Sweet potato, 1 medium	152
Tangerine, 1 medium	40
Tea, 1 bag	1
Tomato, 1 medium	26
Tomato, canned, ½ cup	25
Tomato juice, ½ cup	23
Tongue, pickled, 1 ounce	76
Tortilla, 1	64
Trout, boned, 4 ounces cooked	125
Tuna, water-packed, 6½-ounce can	240
Turkey, roasted, 2 ounces sliced	108
Turnip, diced, ½ cup	18
Turnip greens, cooked, ½ cup	14
Turtle meat, 2 ounces cooked	60
Vanilla extract, 1 teaspoon	8
Veal chop, 4 ounces lean, cooked	220
Veal loin, roasted, 2 ounces	135
Vinegar, 1 tablespoon	2
Waffles, 7-inch diameter, 1	210
Walnuts, ½ cup shelled	326
Water chestnuts, 2 ounces	36
Watercress, ½ cup	3
Watermelon, ½ cup	21
Wheat germ, 1 ounce	103
Whitefish, 4 ounces baked	177
Whitefish, smoked, 4 ounces	177
Yeast, compressed, 1 ounce	25
Yeast, dry, 1 tablespoon	23
Yogurt, skim, plain ½ cup	62
Beer, 12 ounces	150
Brandy, flavored, 1 ounce	75
Champagne, 3 ounces	75
Distilled liquors, 80 proof, 1 ounce	65
Distilled liquors, 100 proof, 1 ounce	82
Wines, dessert, 3 ounces	120
Wines, dry red, 3 ounces	88
Wines, dry white, 3 ounces	75

Appendix B

Instructions for Participating in the Rotation Diet Follow-up Study

You can participate in the Rotation Diet follow-up study by writing to:

The Rotation Diet
c/o The Vanderbilt Weight Management Program
134 Wesley Hall
Vanderbilt University
Nashville, TN 37240

Please indicate specifically that you want to participate in the Rotation Diet follow-up study, *and be sure to include your name and address in your letter.* You will hear from us periodically, at which time we will want to know how you are doing in managing your weight. We will be asking you to fill out a very short questionnaire each time we write to you.

There is no charge for participating in this follow-up study and you will receive no solicitation for anything but information about how well you are doing in managing your weight.

HOW TO OBTAIN MORE INFORMATION ABOUT THE VANDERBILT WEIGHT MANAGEMENT PROGRAM

The Vanderbilt Weight Management Program offers consultation via mail and telephone on weight-management problems.

If you would like to receive information about the consultation services and other weight-management materials that are available at a modest cost from the program, *please send a stamped, self-addressed envelope requesting this information to:*

Associate Director
Vanderbilt Weight Management Program
134 Wesley Hall
Vanderbilt University
Nashville, TN 37240

Please write (rather than call) to obtain this additional information on our consultation services.

The Rotation Diet Pocket Edition for Women

You can average a weight loss of up to a pound a day for twenty-one days if you follow the menus exactly as they are laid out on pages 238–242. Best results are obtained *with no substitutions*. However, if a particular food does not agree with you, please read Chapter 6 concerning allowable substitutions.

Recipes and other suggestions for food preparation are found in Chapter 6. I have not given the names of specific recipes here, as I did in the Chapter 6 menus, but those foods with an asterisk have recipes in Chapter 6.

In order to be sure that everyone can follow the Rotation Diet and never feel hungry, I have designed an insurance policy that will enable you to overcome temptations and still achieve close-to-optimum results. It has two clauses. The first is called *free vegetables*. Should any temptations to deviate from the diet arise during the next twenty-one days, you may eat unlimited quantities of free vegetables with any meal and at any time of the day as snacks (see page 243 of this Pocket Edition). Free vegetables contain almost no calories. In addition, you may choose a *safe fruit* (see page 243 of this Pocket Edition). The safe fruit (remember to choose only one) will be additional insurance against ever being hungry. It will also be used as a source of quick energy whenever you need it.

You may photocopy the Pocket Edition of the Rotation Diet so that you can carry it with you for ready reference. In case a photocopier is not available to you, you may cut out the Pocket Edition pages without damaging the other contents of the book.

COUPLES CAN USE THE ROTATION DIET TOGETHER

See the text at the beginning of the Pocket Edition menus for women (Weeks 1 and 2), or see page 45 of Chapter 6.

> If you show the Rotation Diet to your friends and they wish to use it, please have them read Chapters 1, 6, and 7 before they start. (Be sure to read these chapters yourself before you start.)

THE COMPLETE ROTATION DIET PLAN MENUS FOR WOMEN

The Rotation Diet is designed to be used with the special recipes that are available for items marked with an asterisk (see Chapter 6 menus for specific names of recipes, or leaf through recipes). However, you can prepare everything in your own way provided you do not use any fat in preparation except where indicated. Also, you can use the portion sizes below as a guide when eating out during this period. *Weights below are all cooked weights.* See Chapter 6 for information on shrinkage to be expected during cooking. No-cal salad dressings can be used at any time, so they are not always indicated. Note: tablespoon and teaspoon measures are level measures.

Week 1

In the case of couples who wish to use the Rotation Diet together, men may use the basic Week 1 diet plan for women with the addition of all of the following each day:

2 more grain servings (bread, cereal, or crackers)
50 percent larger portions of meat, fish, or fowl
1 tablespoon of butter, oil, or regular salad dressing
3 safe fruits

The calorie goal for men is 1200 calories for the first three days, and 1500 calories for the next four. Additional information on serving sizes, *with calorie values,* will be found with the recipes in Chapter 6.

DAY 1

Breakfast: ½ grapefruit, 1 slice of whole-wheat bread,* 1 ounce of cheese, no-cal beverage

Lunch: 2 ounces of salmon* (canned in water), unlimited free vegetables, 5 whole-wheat crackers, no-cal beverage

Dinner: 3 ounces of baked chicken,* 1 cup of cauliflower,* ½ cup of beets,* 1 apple, no-cal beverage

DAY 2

Breakfast: ½ banana, 1 ounce of high-fiber cereal,* 8 ounces of skim or low-fat milk, no-cal beverage

Lunch: 4 ounces of low-fat cottage cheese,* unlimited free vegetables, 1 slice of whole-wheat bread,* no-cal beverage

Dinner: 3 ounces of poached fish fillet,* 1 cup of broccoli,* ½ cup of carrots,* ½ grapefruit, no-cal beverage

DAY 3

Breakfast: 1 slice of whole-wheat bread,* 1 tablespoon of peanut butter, 1 apple, no-cal beverage

Lunch: 2 ounces of water-packed tuna* or 3 medium sardines,* 5 whole-wheat crackers, unlimited free vegetables, no-cal beverage

Dinner: 3 ounces of beefsteak* or hamburger patty,* 1 cup of asparagus,* 1 cup of dinner salad,* 1 ounce of cheese, 1 orange, no-cal beverage

DAY 4

Breakfast: ½ banana, 1 ounce of high-fiber cereal,* 8 ounces of skim or low-fat milk, no-cal beverage

Lunch: Tuna salad* (2 ounces of water-packed tuna), unlimited free vegetables, 2 slices of whole-wheat bread,* 1 teaspoon of mayonnaise or lo-cal dressing,* ½ grapefruit, no-cal beverage

Dinner: 3 ounces of baked chicken,* ½ cup of carrots,* 1 cup of dinner salad,* 1 ounce of cheese, 1 apple, no-cal beverage

DAY 5

Breakfast: 1 cup of berries, 4 ounces of low-fat cottage cheese,* 5 whole-wheat crackers, no-cal beverage

Lunch: 3 medium sardines* or 2 ounces of water-packed tuna,* unlimited free vegetables, 2 slices of whole-wheat bread,* 1 teaspoon of mayonnaise or lo-cal dressing,* ½ grapefruit, no-cal beverage

Dinner: 3 ounces of beefsteak* or hamburger patty,* ½ cup of green beans,* 1 cup of broccoli,* 1 ounce of cheese, 1 apple, no-cal beverage

DAY 6

Breakfast: ½ cantaloupe, 1 ounce of cheese, 1 slice of whole-wheat bread,* no-cal beverage

Lunch: 1 hard-boiled egg,* unlimited free vegetables, 2 slices of whole-wheat bread,* 1 teaspoon of mayonnaise or lo-cal salad dressing,* ½ grapefruit, no-cal beverage

Dinner: 3 ounces of fish fillet,* 1 cup of asparagus,* ½ cup of green peas,* 1 apple, no-cal beverage

DAY 7

Breakfast: ½ banana, 1 ounce of high-fiber cereal,* 8 ounces of skim or low-fat milk, no-cal beverage
Lunch: 1 cup of berries, 4 ounces of low-fat cottage cheese,* 2 slices of whole-wheat bread,* no-cal beverage
Dinner: 3 ounces of baked chicken,* 1 cup of cauliflower,* ½ cup of carrots,* 1 apple, no-cal beverage

Week 2

In Week 2 you may add a mid-morning, a mid-afternoon, and an evening snack, intentionally incorporating three servings of your *safe fruit.* It is not obligatory to include all of these snacks in addition to the menus below, but they are permitted within the 1200-calorie limits for this week. You may also add 1 tablespoon of butter, margarine, oil, or regular salad dressing to your diet each day. Use it for cooking or as a spread.

For couples' use, men should add all of the following each day to the daily menus of the Rotation Diet for women, below.

2 more grain servings (bread, cereal, or crackers)
50 percent larger portions of vegetables and main courses

Optional for men: another tablespoon of fat for spread or seasoning. The calorie goal for males is 1800 per day throughout Week 2. Additional information on serving sizes, *with calorie values,* will be found with the recipes in Chapter 6.

DAY 8

Breakfast: ½ grapefruit, 1 slice of whole-wheat bread,* 1 tablespoon of peanut butter, 8 ounces of skim or low-fat milk, no-cal beverage
Lunch: large fruit salad (2 cups),* 1 ounce of cheese, 5 whole-wheat crackers, no-cal beverage
Dinner: salmon steak* (4½ ounces), ½ cup of peas and baby onions,* 1 cup of dinner salad,* no-cal beverage

DAY 9

Breakfast: ½ banana, 1 ounce of high-fiber cereal,* 8 ounces of skim or low-fat milk, no-cal beverage

Lunch: large chef salad* (1 ounce of turkey and 1 ounce of cheese, plus salad vegetables), 5 whole-wheat crackers, lo-cal dressing,* no-cal beverage

Dinner: 4½ ounces of baked chicken,* 1 small (3½-ounce) baked potato, 1 cup of green beans,* 1 ounce of cheese, 1 apple, no-cal beverage

DAY 10

Breakfast: 1 cup of sliced fruit, 4 ounces of low-fat cottage cheese,* 1 slice of whole-wheat bread,* no-cal beverage

Lunch: sandwich* (2 ounces of meat or cheese), unlimited free vegetables, 1 orange, no-cal beverage

Dinner: 2 cups of stir-fry vegetables,* ½ cup of brown or wild rice,* 2 tablespoons of grated cheese, 1 apple, no-cal beverage

DAY 11

Breakfast: 1 cup of fresh pineapple (or other fresh fruit), 1 ounce of cheese, 1 slice of whole-wheat bread,* no-cal beverage

Lunch: large (2–3 cups) spinach salad,* lo-cal dressing,* 1 apple or pear, 1 ounce of cheese, no-cal beverage

Dinner: 6 ounces of steak,* 1 small (3½-ounce) baked potato, 1 cup of braised carrots and celery,* ½ grapefuit, no-cal beverage

DAY 12

Breakfast: ½ cup of sliced fruit for cereal, 1 ounce of high-fiber cereal,* 8 ounces of skim or low-fat milk, no-cal beverage

Lunch: tuna or sardine salad* (3 ounces of water-packed

tuna, 4–5 medium sardines), unlimited free vegetables plus sliced tomato and green peppers, lo-cal dressing,* 1 slice of whole-wheat bread,* no-cal beverage

Dinner: 6 ounces of lean pork chop* (or other lean meat), ½ baked acorn squash,* 1 cup of broccoli,* ½ grapefruit, no-cal beverage

DAY 13

Breakfast: ½ melon, 1 hard- or soft-boiled egg,* 1 slice of whole-wheat bread,* no-cal beverage

Lunch: 4½-ounce ground-beef patty,* 4 ounces of low-fat cottage cheese,* sliced tomato and unlimited free vegetables, lo-cal dressing,* no-cal beverage

Dinner: 1 cup of pasta* (choice of sauces*), 2 tablespoons of Parmesan cheese, 1 cup of dinner salad,* choice of 1 fresh fruit for dessert, no-cal beverage

DAY 14

Breakfast: ½ grapefruit, 1 cup of oatmeal, 2 tablespoons of raisins, dash of cinnamon, 4 ounces of skim or low-fat milk, no-cal beverage

Lunch: toasted open-faced sandwich* or regular sandwich* (2 ounces of meat or cheese), unlimited free vegetables, 1 cup of assorted sliced fresh fruit, no-cal beverage

Dinner: Pot roast of beef* (4 ounces of meat, plus vegetables), 1 cup of dinner salad,* lo-cal dressing,* 1 ounce of cheese, 1 apple, no-cal beverage

Week 3

Repeat the menus of Week 1, or use the Alternate Menus in Chapter 12 for the 600- and 900-calorie rotations.

When you finish your twenty-one days on the Rotation Diet, BE VERY SURE THAT YOU FOLLOW MY DIRECTIONS FOR MAKING A TRANSITION TO MAINTENANCE IN WEEK 4 (CHAPTER 8).

Unlimited Free Vegetable List

You may eat all you want of the vegetables on this list at any time. They provide many vitamins and minerals, together with beneficial amounts of fiber, with virtually no calories. Eat them plain or use only no-cal salad dressings (your choice, or see page 75 of the Rotation Diet).

asparagus	endive	radish
celery	escarole	spinach
chicory	lettuce	watercress
Chinese cabbage	parsley	zucchini
cucumber		

Safe Fruit List

Choose *one* fruit from this list (or any other fresh fruit that is easily available to you) as your *safe fruit*. Eat up to three servings a day in addition to whatever is called for in the menus of the Rotation Diet when you need a lift, feel intolerably hungry, or are tempted to deviate from your diet for any reason. Carry one with you at all times as a snack.

apple	melon	pineapple
berries	orange	tangerine
grapefruit	peach	

Whenever you are tempted to deviate from the Rotation Diet make a safe-fruit substitution instead. This ensures that you will achieve close to the maximum possible weight loss.

Beverages

Drink eight 8-ounce glasses of water a day. Use only no-calorie beverages except when milk is called for. You may drink up to 2 cups of coffee or tea each day, plus herb teas and low-sodium bouillons.

The Rotation Diet
Pocket Edition
for Men

You can average a weight loss of up to a pound a day for twenty-one days if you follow the menus exactly as they are laid out on pages 247–251. Best results are obtained *with no substitutions*. However, if a particular food does not agree with you, please read Chapter 6 concerning allowable substitutions.

Recipes and other suggestions for food preparation are found in Chapter 6. I have not given the names of specific recipes here, as I did in the Chapter 6 menus, but those foods with an asterisk have recipes in Chapter 6.

In order to be sure that everyone can follow the Rotation Diet and never feel hungry, I have designed an insurance policy that will enable you to overcome temptations and still achieve close-to-optimum results. It has two clauses. The first is called *free vegetables*. Should any temptations to deviate from the diet arise during the next twenty-one days, you may eat unlimited quantities of free vegetables with any meal and at any time of the day as snacks (see page 251 of this Pocket Edition). Free vegetables contain almost no calories. In addition, you may choose a *safe fruit* (see page 252 of this Pocket Edition). The safe fruit (remember to choose only one) will be another insur-

ance against ever being hungry. It will also be used as a source
of quick energy whenever you need it.

You may photocopy the Pocket Edition of the Rotation Diet
so that you can carry it with you for ready reference. In case a
photocopier is not available to you, you may cut out the Pocket
Edition pages without damaging the other contents of the book.

COUPLES CAN USE THE ROTATION DIET TOGETHER

See the text at the beginning of the Pocket Edition menus for
women (Weeks 1 and 2), or see page 45 of Chapter 6.

> If you show the Rotation Diet to your friends and they
> wish to use it, please have them read Chapter 1, 6, and
> 7 before they start. (Be sure to read these chapters
> yourself before you start.)

THE COMPLETE ROTATION DIET PLAN MENUS FOR MEN

The Rotation Diet is designed to be used with the special recipes
that are available for items marked with an asterisk (see Chapter
6 menus for specific names of recipes, or leaf through recipes).
However, you can prepare everything in your own way provided
you do not use any fat in preparation except where indicated.
Also, you can use the portion sizes below as a guide when eating
out during this period. *Weights below are all cooked weights.*
See Chapter 6 for information on shrinkage to be expected
during cooking.

Men may add 1 tablespoon of butter, margarine, or regular
salad dressing to each day's menu and remain within the calorie
limits. No-cal salad dressings can be used at any time, so they
are not always indicated.

Men may also plan on having three *safe fruit* snacks each

day, in addition to the items on the following menus. You do not have to eat them all, but they are available, within the calorie limits. Note: tablespoon and teaspoon measures are level measures.

Week 1

DAY 1

Breakfast: ½ banana, 1 ounce of high-fiber cereal,* 8 ounces of skim or low-fat milk, no-cal beverage

Lunch: large chef salad* 1 ounce each of cheese and turkey, plus any salad vegetables), lo-cal dressing,* 5 whole-wheat crackers, no-cal beverage

Dinner: 4½ ounces of baked chicken,* 1 small (3½-ounce) baked potato, 1 cup of green beans,* 1 apple, 1 ounce of cheese, no-cal beverage

DAY 2

Breakfast: ½ grapefruit, 1 slice of whole-wheat bread,* 1 tablespoon of peanut butter, 8 ounces of skim or low-fat milk, no-cal beverage

Lunch: large fruit salad* (2 cups), 1 ounce of cheese, 5 whole-wheat crackers, no-cal beverage

Dinner: 6 ounces of fish fillets,* ½ cup of green peas and baby onions,* 1 cup of dinner salad,* lo-cal dressing,* no-cal beverage

DAY 3

Breakfast: 1 cup of sliced fruit (your choice), 4 ounces of low-fat cottage cheese,* 1 slice of whole-wheat bread,* no-cal beverage

Lunch: combination sandwich* (2 ounces of meat or cheese), unlimited free vegetables, 1 orange, no-cal beverage

Dinner: 2 cups of stir-fry vegetables,* ½ cup of brown or wild rice,* 2 tablespoons of grated cheese, 1 apple, no-cal beverage

DAY 4

Breakfast: 1 cup of berries, 1½ ounces of high-fiber cereal,* 8 ounces of skim or low-fat milk, 1 slice of whole-wheat bread,* 1 teaspoon of preserves, no-cal beverage

Lunch: large (2–3 cups) spinach salad,* lo-cal dressing,* 5 whole-wheat crackers, 1 apple or pear, no-cal beverage

Dinner: ½ grapefruit, 6 ounces of steak,* 1 small (3½-ounce) baked potato, 1 cup of braised carrots and celery,* no-cal beverage

DAY 5

Breakfast: ½ melon, 1 hard- or soft-boiled egg, 2 slices of whole-wheat bread,* 1 teaspoon of preserves, no-cal beverage

Lunch: 4½-ounces ground-beef patty,* 4 ounces of low-fat cottage cheese,* unlimited free vegetables, 1 slice of whole-wheat bread,* 1 serving of fruit (your choice), no-cal beverage

Dinner: 1 cup of pasta* (choice of sauces*), 4 tablespoons of Parmesan cheese, 1 cup of dinner salad,* lo-cal dressing,* ½ grapefruit, no-cal beverage

DAY 6

Breakfast: 1 cup of sliced fruit, 1½ ounces of high-fiber cereal,* 1 slice of whole-wheat bread, 8 ounces of skim or low-fat milk, no-cal beverage

Lunch: sardine or tuna salad* (4–5 medium sardines or 3 ounces of water-packed tuna), unlimited free vegetables plus sliced tomato and green pepper, lo-cal dressing,* 2 slices of whole-wheat bread,* no-cal beverage

Dinner: 6 ounces of lean pork chop* (or other lean meat*), baked acorn squash,* 1 cup of broccoli,* 1 slice of whole-wheat bread,* ½ grapefruit, no-cal beverage

DAY 7

Breakfast: ½ grapefruit, 1 cup of oatmeal, 2 tablespoons of raisins, dash of cinnamon, 4 ounces of skim or low-fat milk, no-cal beverage

Lunch: open-faced sandwich* (2 portions, see Mexican Bean Spread,* with 1 ounce of cheese and sliced tomato, or see lunch sandwich Day 3), unlimited free vegetables, lo-cal dressing,* 1 cup of assorted fresh fruit, no-cal beverage

Dinner: 4 ounces of pot roast* (including vegetables), 1 cup of dinner salad,* lo-cal dressing,* 1 apple, no-cal beverage

Week 2

DAY 8

Breakfast: ½ melon, 2 slices of whole-wheat bread,* 2 ounces of cheese, no-cal beverage

Lunch: tuna-salad sandwich* (3 ounces of water-packed tuna), unlimited free vegetables, 1 serving of fruit (your choice), no-cal beverage

Dinner: 6 ounces of baked chicken,* ½ cup of spinach and broccoli casserole* (or 1 cup of broccoli*), ½ baked acorn squash,* 1 apple, 1 ounce of cheese (if casserole recipe is not used), no-cal beverage

DAY 9

Breakfast: 1 cup of oatmeal, 2 tablespoons of raisins, dash of cinnamon, 4 ounces of skim or low-fat milk, 1 slice of whole-wheat bread,* 1 teaspoon of preserves, no-cal beverage

Lunch: large fruit salad* (2 cups), 4 ounces of low-fat cottage cheese,* 5 whole-wheat crackers, no-cal beverage

Dinner: 6 ounces of fish fillet,* ½ baked tomato,* 1 small (3½-ounce) baked potato, 1 cup of dinner salad,* 1 ounce of cheese, 1 apple, no-cal beverage

DAY 10

Breakfast: 1 orange, 2 slices of whole-wheat bread,* 2 ounces of cheese, no-cal beverage

Lunch: tuna salad* (3 ounces of water-packed tuna) on greens with sliced tomatoes and green pepper, plus unlimited free vegetables, lo-cal dressing,* no-cal beverage

Dinner: 6 ounces of steak,* 1 cup of stir-fry spinach,* 1 small (3½-ounce) baked potato with cottage-cheese dressing* (or 2 tablespoons of sour cream), choice of 1 fruit, no-cal beverage

DAY 11

Breakfast: ½ melon, 4 ounces of low-fat cottage cheese,* 1 slice of whole-wheat bread,* 1 teaspoon of preserves, no-cal beverage

Lunch: sandwich* (2 ounces of meat or cheese), unlimited free vegetables, lo-cal dressing,* no-cal beverage

Dinner: 6 ounces of baked salmon,* ½ cup of peas and baby onions,* 1 cup of dinner salad,* lo-cal dressing,* choice of 1 fruit, 1 ounce of cheese, no-cal beverage

DAY 12

Breakfast: ½ grapefruit, 2 slices of whole-wheat bread,* 1 tablespoon of peanut butter, 1 teaspoon of preserves, no-cal beverage

Lunch: 1 cup of soup (commercial or see Soups*), 10 whole-wheat crackers, 2 ounces of cheese, unlimited free vegetables, lo-cal dressing,* no-cal beverage

Dinner: veal loaf* (or 6-ounce serving of lean meat of your choice*), ½ cup of carrots,* 1 cup of dinner salad,* lo-cal dressing,* 1 apple, no-cal beverage

DAY 13

Breakfast: 1 cup of berries, 1½ ounces of high-fiber cereal,* 1 slice of whole-wheat bread,* 1 teaspoon of preserves, 8 ounces of skim or low-fat milk, no-cal beverage

Lunch: large chef salad* (1 ounce each of turkey and cheese, plus salad vegetables), lo-cal dressing,* 5 whole-wheat crackers, no-cal beverage

Dinner: 6 ounces of baked chicken,* ½ cup of brown or wild rice,* 1 cup of broccoli,* 1 ounce of cheese, 1 apple, no-cal beverage

DAY 14

Breakfast: 1 cup of sliced fruit, 4 ounces of low-fat cottage cheese,* 1 slice of whole-wheat bread,* 1 teaspoon of preserves, no-cal beverage

Lunch: sandwich* (2 ounces of meat or cheese), unlimited free vegetables, lo-cal dressing,* ½ grapefruit, no-cal beverage

Dinner: 6 ounces of baked or broiled fish,* ½ baked tomato,* 1 cup of green beans with chives,* 1 slice of whole-wheat bread,* 1 ounce of cheese, 1 fruit of your choice, no-cal beverage

Week 3

Repeat the menus of Week 1, or use the Alternate Menus in Chapter 12 for the 1200- and 1500-calorie rotations.

When you finish your twenty-one days on the Rotation Diet, BE VERY SURE THAT YOU FOLLOW MY DIRECTIONS FOR MAKING A TRANSITION TO MAINTENANCE IN WEEK 4 (CHAPTER 8).

Unlimited Free Vegetable List

You may eat all you want of the vegetables in this list at any time. They provide many vitamins and minerals, together with beneficial amounts of fiber, with virtually no calories. Eat them plain or use only no-cal salad dressings (your choice, or see page 75 of the Rotation Diet).

asparagus	endive	radish
celery	escarole	spinach
chicory	lettuce	watercress
Chinese cabbage	parsley	zucchini
cucumber		

Safe Fruit List

Choose *one* fruit from this list (or any other fresh fruit that is easily available to you) as your *safe fruit*. Eat up to three servings a day in addition to whatever is called for in the menus of the Rotation Diet when you need a lift, feel intolerably hungry, or are tempted to deviate from your diet for any reason. Carry one with you at all times as a snack.

apple	melon	pineapple
berries	orange	tangerine
grapefruit	peach	

Whenever you are tempted to deviate from the Rotation Diet make a safe-fruit substitution instead. This ensures that you will achieve close to the maximum possible weight loss.

Beverages

Drink eight 8-ounce glasses of water a day. Use only no-calorie beverages except when milk is called for. You may drink up to 2 cups of coffee or tea each day, plus herb teas and low-sodium bouillons.

Index

Boldfaced page numbers refer to recipes.